GIFTS OF H

MICHAEL HARPER, a medical doctor, is the Director of Burrswood Hospital and Place of Healing. Founded by Dorothy Kerin in 1948, it provides Christian prayer for healing as well as practical care for unwell people – the marriage of ministry and medicine, of care and prayer. In this identity, it remains unique.

MICHAEL FULLJAMES, an Anglican priest, recently retired as the Chaplain of Burrswood. He now lives in Canterbury.

GIFTS
OF HEALING

Prayers for those who
care for the sick

MICHAEL HARPER
and
MICHAEL FULLJAMES

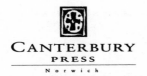

CANTERBURY
PRESS
Norwich

© Michael Fulljames and Michael Harper 2005

First published in 2005 by
the Canterbury Press Norwich
(a publishing imprint of
Hymns Ancient & Modern Limited,
a registered charity)
St Mary's Works, St Mary's Plain,
Norwich, Norfolk, NR3 3BH

www.scm-canterburypress.co.uk

British Library Cataloguing in Publication data

A catalogue record for this book is available
from the British Library

ISBN 1-85311-639-4/9781-85311-639-1

Typeset by Regent Typesetting, London
Printed and bound in Great Britain by Bookmarque Ltd

CONTENTS

INTRODUCTION

We have observed in our careers in medicine and ministry the remarkable ways in which the disaster of illness affects people, and realized that there is indeed something profoundly redemptive about it. We have sat with the afflicted and heard their cries. We have prayed with them in their need, laughed with them in their joy at being healed and, at times, wept when that healing has not been forthcoming. We have realised that God is indeed 'past finding out'. Sometimes we simply don't understand; but we have enough experience of God to hold us steady in the extent of the valley of doubt to which we have thus far been exposed.

But we have seen, within the whole drama of illness, unsung heroes, and this book is for them. They are the carers. They too wrestle, and fight, and pray, and try, and they too sometimes fail. The pressures upon them can be enormous. The late Dame Cicely Saunders, founder of St Christopher's Hospice, has reminded us that the burden of care is independent of any work done – just to have primary responsibility is a great burden. Carers, we have watched you; we salute you; and we hope that this small volume will encourage you at least a little.

And we have tried to allow our thoughts to embrace professional carers as well, for caring as a job is demanding, difficult and at times discouraging. Whether you are a nurse, doctor, pastor, counsellor, therapist or social worker: may you, too, find a little encouragement within these pages.

We want to thank our wives, Kitty and Jane; they have put up with endless 'absences' over the months with wonderful grace and generosity, and still encouraged us! Thank you. And we also wish to record our gratitude to Christine Smith and Mary Matthews, of Canterbury Press, who have tolerated our tardiness with great grace; and advised and encouraged us in this little adventure with wisdom and discernment. Thank you.

Michael and Michael

GIFTS
OF HEALING

CALLED TO CARE

*I have read in Plato and Cicero sayings that
are very wise and very beautiful; but I never
read in either of them 'Come unto me all ye
that labour and are heavy laden'.*

St Augustine of Hippo, AD 354–430

Some know they have been called to be
carers, as a vocation.

Others just find themselves cast in that
role.

All discover that it's often not easy: in fact,
sometimes it's extremely demanding.

Often it engages us to the point where our
liberty is restricted – especially in looking
after a family member . . .

And there is that burden of responsibility before a finger is lifted. The late Dame
Cicely Saunders described this as a great
burden – not the care, but just having the
responsibility for the one to be cared for.
Practical aspects of caring only add to that
burden.

*Do what you can,
With what you
have,
Where you are.*
T. Roosevelt
(1851–1919)

Professional carers can find themselves
doing more than a fulltime job.

It extends into overtime, worry-time and
even dream-time.

And some can find resentment creeping
in . . .

At times I have been tempted to put a
notice on my surgery door – 'Please only

*I do not pray for
a lighter load, but
a stronger back.*
Philip Brookes
(1835–95)

come in if you're feeling worse than me!'
But I can't.

A 'child' near three score years and ten
finds herself worn out looking after Mum;
she's 95, and doesn't miss a beat. Then
her husband gets sick, and she falls into
despair. It happens.

Being a carer can be really tough.

What emotions can we feel?

Yes, joy at the privilege of caring.

But also, at times, guilt, desperation, exhaustion, worry, anger, resentment.

Even bitterness at the lowest times: 'Why
me?'

We need help.

We need the understanding of others.

*The experience of
the whole gamut
of emotions is a
part of the human
condition, the
inheritance of
every man.*
John Powell, SJ

We need the help of God, and we need to
feel his love.

Perhaps it all starts with just getting a
glimpse of God's special love for these
who care in his name.

For it is his work they do, his love they
reflect, and they carry a cross as surely as
Jesus carried his. A bit smaller, yes; but still
a cross.

We, the two Michaels, find ourselves praying especially for you as a carer, that you
may know his love in your heart, whether
it be as a 'professional', or as a family member – because you need it, and sometimes
no one quite understands how much; and
we pray that this little book of meditations
and prayers will strengthen you and encourage you day by day.

CALLED TO CARE

O give thanks to the Lord, call on his name,
make known his deeds among the peoples.
Sing to him, sing praises to him; tell of all his
wonderful works.

Psalm 105.1–2

Lord of all life, Lord of all love, Lord of all
truth:
Thanks and praise and glory be to you;
You know each of us, you seek us and you
call us.

Lord of all life, aware of us from the very
beginning:
We thank you, for you called us by name;
prepare us to know your promises and
purposes.

Lord of all truth, knowing our gifts and
potential:
We praise you for opening our eyes to your
plans; by your spirit you stir our ears to
answer your call.

Lord of all love, calling us close – into
your presence: we glorify you; your works
are plain to our view; open our hearts to
respond to your desires.

*Seek the Lord
and his strength;
seek his presence
continually.*
Psalm 105.4

Lord of all comfort, Lord of all wisdom, Lord of all grace: pray give us your courage and your persistence on the days we don't feel up to this calling.

Lord of all wisdom, understanding what it is to be on one's own: pray grant us your counsel and discernment when the day looks foggy and confusing.

Lord of all grace, pray help us with your presence and sharing, each step of the way, and even to the end of time; strengthen us when the cross feels so heavy.

*The steadfast love
of the Lord never
ceases, his mercies
never come to an
end;
They are new every
morning: Great is
your faithfulness.*
Lamentations
3.22–23

Lord of all power, Lord of all wonder, Lord of all faithfulness: alleluia – for those days when the cross we took up becomes that yoke you promised would feel light.

Lord of all wonder, open our eyes to see your transformation: alleluia – for those days when our sighs and blunders become your amazing signs and wonders.

Lord of all faithfulness, trusting us with your precious works: alleluia – for you call us to do in your name works that can give bright glimpses of glory.

Alleluia,
Alleluia,
Alleluia.

INSPIRATION

> *Come, Holy Ghost, our souls inspire, and lighten with*
> *celestial fire;*
> *thou the anointing Spirit art, who dost thy sevenfold*
> *gifts impart.*

In the traditional healing service at the Burrswood Christian Centre as this ancient hymn, 'Veni Creator Spiritus', is sung by the congregation the ministers pray over each other to be healed, prepared and inspired for their ministry.

One then feels really strengthened and encouraged to exercise the ministry to which one is called. We readily think of clinical and pastoral works as vocations, we enter our work with enthusiasm; it is not just a job. We may feel inspired, or seek inspiration so that we can increase in devotion and commitment on behalf of those we serve. We would probably readily agree that it is only later that we comprehend the full meaning of what this is all about; and then discover the limits that the real world would try to put on our idealism.

Very many carers, however, have virtually no choice as to whether it is a vocation in which they find themselves. Thoughts of inspiration will be one of the last things on our minds and hearts, as we slip into or are plunged into a seriously challenging caring role at home. However the circumstances arise, what calls for attention are very practical and heavy tasks. The voice that calls is that of a needy loved one, which may well seem to clamour more loudly than the still, quiet voice of God. There may be little pause to reflect on what is happening, emotionally and spiritually, within the day-to-day caring routines, and in the struggle to gain the support and help needed from sources outside the home.

What such devoted and committed carers are offering are practical works of mercy, whether they would use the word or not. To think of inspiration as merely a spiritual matter in these circumstances may miss the point. What gives the energy and strength to meet the demands of the caring role? When supportive friends are able to lend a hand, to share – then we know the feeling of being lifted, a buzz, a renewal of enthusiasm.

The Holy Spirit inspires as much in the practical body as in the soul. Sadly, Church people are not always very good at this. In his book, *Trust Me, I'm a Carer* (found at www. Imacarer.co.uk), John Brooks writes an evocative chapter, 'Priests, Levites and Samaritans', showing the difficulties faithful people had in facing what had happened after his wife's stroke. They were thus mostly unable to reach beyond the Churchy and 'Spiritual'.

Surely we need something over and above normal human imagination. In times of dreariness we need Holy Spirit-filled energy and insight; to be set free to be courageous and bold, and fulfil God's merciful purposes. Jesus renewed his energy and vitality. Early morning prayer enabled him: to renew his strength, to rise up like an eagle, to run and not be weary, to walk and not faint (paraphrase Isaiah 40.31).

Finding strength in our communion with the Lord, we can pray for his divine love – the energy which is as practical and useful as grace, mercy and peace.

INSPIRATION

I need inspiration, Lord. I need whatever will keep me strong, faithful and seeing the point of everything – as far as that is possible.

Yes, I think I need people, but I also need you; and I need to see things through your eyes. Yes.

He who wants a great deal must not ask for a little.
Italian proverb

I want to rise up like an eagle, and feel your presence, and look down from your vantage point.
I want to feel the up-draught of your Spirit lifting me higher – higher – higher,
into your presence, into that place where the things I have to do day after dreary day fall away, and my whole vision is filled with beauty. Your beauty and the true beauty of the one I care for.

As it is, I'm afraid it's bodily fluids that all too often dominate. I sympathize with the one who said, 'I don't do bodily fluids.'
I wonder why you made the very ones you wanted to be like you in your beauty
so appallingly messy.
Bodies are fine when the owners are in control; but when they're not, I find the design wanting.

So, inspire me, O Lord my God!
Let me see your beauty; then let me see the
beauty of this one I am caring for;
the beauty of the person inside the shell.
Please: let me see this one as you do.

And would you send a Samaritan to encourage me? – because I need real human
inspiration too; someone caring, practical
and loving.
Please keep the Levites and Pharisees
away.
Just give me one godly Samaritan for an
hour or two three times a week – one with
a sense of humour too, please, to help me
regain mine.

Lord, I fear, lest my attitudes might rob me
of your presence.
Keep me sweet; keep me genuinely caring,
wholeheartedly loving.
And keep me worshipping you with all my
being.
Inspire me, and send your servants who
will do the same, I pray.

Amen.

GIVING OUT

> *For there were many coming and going, and
> (the apostles) did not even have time to eat.*
>
> Mark 6.31b

Who cares for ME?
Caring can so easily be one big giving out:
expiration without inspiration.
We carry caring like a load; light it is not,
and its weight increases with our weariness.
And in our weaker moments, even a small
task needing doing dominates our perspective, persuading us that it is great of
itself.
It is not.
But it has caught us; the demand dominates and our freedom is robbed.

*My life is draining
away, and my
substance being
sucked dry.*

Anatole Broyard

Yet we are plagued by a pervading guilt
and feeling of selfishness as soon as we
indulge such thoughts.

Most can care for a while.
But caring is rather like pain; the burden
of it is linked both to its intensity and how
long it goes on.
We all bear pain if we perceive it as
temporary.
But chronic pain which seems never to
end? – for that the threshold of tolerance
is much lower.

*And he said,
'Come aside by
yourselves to a
deserted place and
rest awhile.'*
Mark 6.31a

Its very chronicity, its unrelenting nature, sensitizes us; and so it is with caring. We get caring fatigue. We go through the motions, but the caring has somehow diminished.

How then might we reverse that change; to care with all our heart again?
Perhaps three ploys might help.

First, to take proper time off regularly. We are not alone; there are others who can care too, and we must let them.
Jesus did it. He knew that coming apart geographically from time to time stopped him coming apart at the seams – for he had the same needs as we.

Second, to care as though it were Christ we serve – for in a real sense it is. 'Insomuch as you did it to one of these little ones, you did it unto me.'

*Christ has no
hands but our
hands to do this
work today.*
Annie Johnson
Flint (1862–1932)

Third, to breathe in of God's Spirit with every breath, and breathe out our frustrations, irritations and resentments; to make each breath a prayer, and to let that, through practice, become a habit. 'Pray without ceasing.'

GIVING OUT

No refuge remains to me; no one cares for me.
I cry to you, O Lord; I say, 'You are my
refuge, my portion in the land of the living.'
Give heed to my cry for I am brought very low.

Psalm 142.4–6

Fatherly God, I am rapidly emptying –
giving out, exhausting my resources,
Here, there and nearly everywhere;
yesterday, today and for how long;
Weariness and weakness are
overcoming me, I confess.

Fatherly God, I need refuge: can I – may I
find refuge in you?
Just sufficient space, Father? Just
enough quiet; time to be still.
I pray, let your calm reach me,
your peace enfold me.

Give ear to my prayer, O God; do not hide yourself from my supplication.
Cast your burden on the Lord, and he will sustain you;
He will never permit the righteous to be moved.
I will trust you.
Psalm 55.1, 22, 23b

Fatherly God, in your arms my agitations
start to melt away;
Your still small voice sounds so very
soothing.
I feel held up, supported, secure,
being refreshed.

Lord Jesus, teacher and friend, I thank
you for your understanding;
You have taught me to come quietly
to the Father,
Even very early in the day, in the
still of the night.

*Humble yourselves
therefore under
the mighty hand
of God, so that he
may exalt you in
due time.
Cast all your cares
on him, for he
cares for you.*
1 Peter 5.6, 7

Lord Jesus, you know what it is like when
everywhere seems quiet,
> But the turmoil in the heart makes
> for a wakeful night.
> > Heal my soul, I cry, through
> > your agony and passion.

Lord Jesus, Master and Redeemer, your
touch renews my spirit.
> I feel your strength, your guidance,
> as I answer your call;
> > To see you, serve you, love you
> > in those for whom I care.

Holy Spirit, Spirit of wisdom and understanding, by your mercy
> May I breathe out the frustrations,
> irritations and resentments.
> > May you breathe into me your
> > holiness and insight.

Anointing Spirit, Spirit of counsel and
inward strength, by your grace

*May the amazing
grace of the
master, Jesus
Christ, the
extravagant love
of God our father,
the intimate
friendship of the
Holy Spirit be
with us all.*
(based on
2 Corinthians
13.14, *The Message*)

> May I learn to seek your space, and
> then pace my days.
> > May you teach me to work only
> > in your power.

Sanctifying Spirit, Spirit of knowledge
and true godliness,
> May I turn my face always – but
> always – towards your love.
> > Then will you cause me to pray
> > without ceasing.

FINDING RESOURCES

*To grow is to emerge gradually from a land where our
vision is limited,
where we are seeking and governed by egotistical pleasure,
by our sympathies and antipathies, to a land of
unlimited horizons and
universal love, where we will be open to every person
and desire their happiness.*

Jean Vanier, founder of the L'arche communities

For the believer, ultimately all the creative power that causes
and sustains growth comes from God. How is this power to
be found, received and used to reach fulfilment and achieve-
ment of purpose? Growth, whether spiritual, personal or
professional is mediated in many ways.

Who am I? How do I grow? My genetic make-up influences
who I become, even how healthy I shall turn out. There
are other social and cultural inheritances that have parts to
play, as does the environment of my upbringing, in both my
physical and emotional aspects. The discovery and joy of
the relationship with God in our spiritual formation will be
of the deepest significance. The ways in which we are able to
relate to others help us blossom, or learn through adversity,
in the interactions that give liveliness or pain. Experience,
education and professional training open up prospects into
the wider world and vocational service.

At this point we discover that 'finding resources', 'professional development' and 'in-service training' suddenly have

a new meaning. By and large this is mostly very valuable –
we are saved from withering in our practice or pastorate,
and our latent gifts are harnessed. It is to the benefit of our
professional performance, and thus our clients.

But though it makes us more competent in a mechanical
professional manner does it all get to the 'heart of me'? When
I consider the me that I am rather than the role in which
I work, what really builds me up? What is it that meets my
need to belong, to be accepted, to have space to make my
choices without feeling pressurized?

We grow best when we are able to take responsibility for our
human needs, and seek to meet them by making relationship. This is as true in the relationship we have with God as
it is of the relationships we have with others, whether they
are our loved ones, our professional peers or those we serve.
It is true even of my very self, for I need to be at peace with
me. It is in exercising relationship that our resources can
blossom.

As we use basic human resources in growing, can we be seeking to reflect the incarnate reality of the one who mended
broken hearts, healed and forgave with no more 'training'
than a carpenter gains at the bench? We stand the same before him, whether we are described with a title of status and
a string of qualifications, or granted the ultimate dignity of
practising sacrificial love as we care in the family home. It
will be in our humanness, with God's love flowing through
us, that we shall discover the gift of our true value. In thus
blessing us, God brings in a valuable harvest.

God does not love us because we are valuable.
We are valuable because God loves us.
Fulton John Sheen

FINDING RESOURCES

*God is so good that He only awaits our desire
to overwhelm us with the gift of Himself.*

Francis Fenelon (1651–1715)

Dear Lord, I'm not sure where the resources I need are to come from.

I suspect I am not alone in feeling that those I have are barely adequate.

*God carries your
picture in His
wallet.*
Tony Campo

Please steer me to the resources you have for me, wherever they may be.

I think about where your resources came from.

Not just from your training, I know.
Much of your training was with wood, which never answers back, is only occasionally awkward, and if it proves excessively so can always be burned for heat.

Yet you always knew what was in a man or a woman, where their 'knots' were, and you were always equal to every situation. And still are.

God hugs you.
Hildegarde of
Bingen
(1098–1179)

Then let me grow in my ability to care not just through training, but through

Who falls for love of God shall rise like a star.
Ben Jonson
(1572–1637)

becoming more like you. Through knowing you, and walking with you.

So I will not despise the training I have received, but nor will I see it as the 'be all and end all'.

Lord, you who give me life, you who give all good gifts, grant me wisdom, patience, love, joy, peace and, when I need it, endurance.

Grant me enough reserves to see the funny side of things, lest I become so serious that people avoid me.

And fill my heart with thanksgiving for all you give me; for all your love and care.

He who laughs – lasts.
Anon.

I want to be a gentle carer, quick to comfort but with twinkly eyes, a quick smile, and a ready laugh.

Yes. Give me what I need to love and laugh, I pray.

HEAL THE SICK

Burrswood is a Christian Healing Centre which incorporates a small hospital. It was founded in 1948 by Dorothy Kerin – a lady with a commission from God. That commission was to heal the sick, comfort the sorrowing and give faith to the faithless.

In my end is my beginning.
Mary Stuart
(1542–87)

Ever since, Burrswood has pursued the path of praying, caring, comforting – a ministry that embraces body, soul and spirit.

Sickness is a mystery. We are born with bodies, and with spirits, and when God breathes into us we become 'a living soul'. The essence of our being transcends the physical; but mortality is the lot of this physical body.

So ministering to the dying is caring at a point of transition.

And seeking God's healing – through both prayer and care – looks to maintaining the unity of body, soul and spirit; it maintains the living in this earthly sphere.

Death is but a path that must be trod
If man would ever pass to God
Thomas Parnell
(1679–1718)

It is a high calling. It presupposes God's will and purpose that the subject of our attention should live. In truth, many of us who care for the sick, seeking their healing, breathe the prayer 'yet not our will, but yours, be done' – for all life in the body will cease.

It is just a matter of when. Lazarus was raised, but died again.

Often we simply do not know what our ministry is achieving – are we the Ananias for a Paul, the Peter for a Dorcas?

Or are we the gentleness of God himself, ministering through the transition that he himself is permitting? – and in which is no disaster?

Death – the last sleep?
No, it is the final awakening.
Sir Walter Scott
(1771–1832)

This gentle resting in the Lord's own purposes for each individual was a key part in Dorothy Kerin's approach to divine healing; but it requires that we submit our all to him, recognizing and resting in his purposes for us and for those we love. She stated it simply in her *Little Way of Prayer*, which we shall visit tonight.

Only by approaching a ministry of healing the sick fully aware of these mysteries, yielded to God's purpose, humble enough to hear, can we truly be his hands to the sick.

Perhaps we might begin by joining our hands with his, and saying – 'Lord, grant that your will in its fullness may be achieved in my work – from the amazing miracle for one to the tender dying care of the other, and all that's in between; you lead, and I will follow.'

HEAL THE SICK

Let us by an act of the will place ourselves in the presence of our Divine Lord, and with an act of faith ask that he will empty us of self and of all desire save that His Most Blessed Will may be done, and that it may illumine our hearts and minds. We can then gather together ourselves and all those for whom our prayers have been asked, and hold all silently up to him, making no special request – neither asking nor beseeching – but just resting, with them, in Him, desiring nothing but that Our Lord may be glorified in all.
Dorothy Kerin
(*A Little Way of Prayer*)

(*The material on this page is taken from, or inspired by, the Burrswood Order of Service for Laying-on-of-Hands, 1989*)

And now, O God, I give myself to Thee.
Empty me of all that is not of Thee,
Cleanse me from all unrighteousness,
And according to Thy will
Take my hands and use them for Thy glory.
Amen

Let us bless the Lord: thanks be to God.

First, O Lord our God, I thank you for who you are: the tender loving merciful God, giver of healing, comfort and faith, in body, mind and spirit; bringing through the touch of Jesus the wholeness that is your desire.

O Lord our God, I thank you for the movement of your Spirit in our time: for the renewal of the Church's ministry of healing; for the wonderful advances in medical science and human understanding; for the inspiration and devotion in all who care for love's sake.

O Lord, I thank you for those many who have known your healing touch upon them, whether triggered by prayer, by clinical intervention or by human compassion. I thank you for the new hope of those who have been released from fear, saved from despair, and delivered from the grip of moments past . . .

O Lord, I thank you for your abundant blessings in many places, for the growth of fellowships and chains of prayer and healing, for the prayers of so many faithful folk, and finally for the life and prayers of those who first interceded for us, for your servant Dorothy Kerin, founder of Burrswood, and for all the Saints.

Lord, hear our prayer; and let our cry come unto thee:

In your presence, Divine Lord, asking in faith that your blessed will may be done, I silently hold up to you:
> Those called to Christ's healing ministry;
> Doctors and Nurses, Therapists and Counsellors, and all who care at home;
> All those being prepared for these and other caring works;
>> that all may enjoy your gifts of boldness, wisdom and humility.
> All who are in hospices and in hospitals, homes of healing and nursing homes,
>> and other centres for therapy and rehabilitation.

Gathering together, Divine Lord, all those for whom my prayers have been asked:
> whether sick or sorrowful, in disturbance or despair, disabled or carrying heavy burdens of care, I lift them to you in the silence of my heart . . .

COMFORT THE SORROWING

Blessed be the God and Father of our Lord Jesus Christ,
the Father of mercies and God of all comfort, who comforts us
in all our affliction,
so that we may be able to comfort those who are in
any affliction,
with the comfort with which we ourselves are comforted by God.

2 Corinthians 1.3, 4

To be a comforter can indeed be difficult. Job's three comforters made a very good start. When they came with condolences to comfort him, they wept and they sat down beside him for seven days saying nothing, seeing how great his suffering was. It was only when they spoke that things started to go wrong.

Have you ever kept silence for an hour, a day, let alone a week with someone in grief? No? Professionally or informally we want to make our intervention. Our world is one that demands action and results. The counsellors among us know how important are patience, taking time, not hurrying and so making space for the inbuilt ability to work through grief.

Much has been learned about the nature and process of people's sorrows; and about the skills needed to stay alongside and be of comforting value to them. The believer can readily see that this is a work and ministry of God. Our introductory text shows we can only be comforters when we have received God's comforting strength ourselves. It implies we must also have learned to express our mourning. Jesus said, 'Blessed are those who mourn, for they shall be comforted' (Matthew 5.4) Only when we let ourselves mourn, without denying or pushing feelings away, are we open to receive the blessing of comfort.

From his own experience of mourning in agony and sorrow in the garden of Gethsemane, Jesus knows our need for comfort.

When he himself has cause for sorrow, and is also the comforter, he shows his humanity in his emotional responses. When he arrives to see Martha and Mary after the death of Lazarus he first suffers the pain of reproach from the mourners and then the delay of theological talk; but touched by the tears of Mary and others he expresses his empathy and compassion. He wept with those who wept. We too should weep with those who weep.

Cath, a Burrswood counsellor, said, 'If you don't cry, you go rusty inside.' Why do so many, especially men, find it so hard to weep with those who weep? To weep is so natural. Are we professionally inhibited, by fear of inappropriate emotional involvement? The funeral could be mayhem if the priest bursts into tears.

For our sorrows Jesus promised the company of the Holy Spirit, 'the Comforter'. He knew whom we needed. With this Spirit alongside us, we shall all find comfort and strength.

COMFORT THE SORROWING

It is always easier if we insulate ourselves from the pain of others.

Yet, as I watch those who seem to be untouched by the sorrow around them, I am sad for them; they are somehow missing so much.
Nonetheless, at times I wish I was like them; I would have more room for my own feelings.

Anyway, all this musing is of little value because, dear Lord, I think you want me to be a comforter.

Sympathy is your pain in my heart.
Anon.

Then teach me to enter fully into the pain of others without becoming overwhelmed. Teach me to weep with those who weep that both of us might be touched and healed, or at least know the beginning of the healing work.

Reach into *my* hurting places, that I might see how *you* comfort once again; model your care in my life – remind me how you do it. And I shall seek to be your disciple and do likewise.

Lord, if I am a disciple (and I want to be),
that makes me a learner.
Then teach me patiently.

Ah. You want to teach me on the job.
You want me just to go ahead and try?
No. You want me to go ahead and start,
and you will give me the words?
How? I see. Your Holy Spirit will tell me
what to say, or what not to say.

*The Holy
Spirit does not
obliterate a man's
personality; he lifts
it to its highest
use.*
Oswald Chambers
(1874–1917)

Forgive me for wondering whether I will
hear him, Lord;
It's just that I feel a little vulnerable.

You know. You know? You know how I
feel? You do!
Hallelujah! – how I am comforted by
that!
That gives me the courage to try; please,
Lord, keep me encouraged
And let your Holy Spirit be the paraklete,
The one who will remain alongside. Thank
you, Lord; I'll try.
I bless you, I worship you; let me be lost in
your love . . .

Yes, and in my lostness, let me bring your
love to others.

GIVE FAITH

Do you believe that I am able to do this?
'Lord, I believe; help Thou my unbelief!'

Mark 9.24

Belief can be astonishingly divorced from any belief system: 'I believe', people say.

Where reason cannot wade, there faith may swim.
Thomas Watson
(1557–92)

But though the desperate father who cried those unforgettable words found in Jesus focus and grounds for his belief, yet actually believing for his son was an agonizing struggle.

The commission given to Dorothy Kerin, founder of Burrswood, has already been quoted in these pages: to heal the sick, comfort the sorrowing and give faith to the faithless – those lacking faith, all in the name of Christ.
It is not a bland, nondescript faith she was commanded to communicate, for that is tantamount to platitude, and in truth of little value to anyone.
It is faith in a God who loves us, and in Jesus Christ who, as God in flesh, came to demonstrate that love, and open the way to heaven.

But how on earth can we 'give faith'? Communicate it to others? We might begin by considering again what happened to give *us* faith, and in what ways it has been successfully stimulated since we first believed.

Faith in Christ is usually born and maintained by a combination of the words and deeds of others who have come into our lives.

But unless words and deeds tally, the chances are we won't believe. We can all too easily spot the hypocrites, and they can terribly easily immunize us against faith for a long time.

But find someone who claims faith and lives differently as a consequence – not in a way that pronounces judgement on all and sundry, or detracts from aliveness, but in an attractive, vibrant way – and we and others listen.

We want to know what makes that one different. We feel loved by that one, and valued – and want the same quality of life.

So how can we communicate faith? Is not this the beginning; to simply be, and then to speak – to let our being authenticate our message?

Yet how hard that can be! How we need to encourage one another!

And then to pray much for those for whom we care. Walk the walk, talk the talk, pray the prayers . . .

GIVE FAITH

Not a burden we bear, not a sorrow we share,
But our toil he doth richly repay;
Not a grief nor a loss, not a frown nor a cross,
but is blest if we trust and obey.
Trust and obey, for there's no better way
To be happy in Jesus, but to trust and obey.

John Henry Sammis (1846–1919)

Glory be to you, all generous God,
> for you gave us life and joy and
> wonder;
Blessings be upon you, ever-loving Father,
> for you gave us your son Jesus;
Thanks be to you, dear Lord Jesus,
> for you gave yourself and your life
> for us;
Praise be to you, most holy Spirit,
> for you stirred up the gift of faith
> in us.

Lord, I trust you, I have confidence in
you;
> yet must I also confess my unbelief,
> moments of wobbliness or doubt,
> times when I do not treasure your
> gift of faith as I should.

Lord, sustain my belief, so that I may not
perish
> but be welcome within eternal life –
> following your way, living your
> truth,
> glad to trust and obey.

Great is thy faithfulness, O God my Father, there is no shadow of turning with Thee; Thou changest not, Thy compassions they fail not, as Thou hast been Thou for ever wilt be.
T. O. Chisholm
(1866–1960)

In your great mercy, Lord, love me still,
    erase my guilt, calm my fears,
    recall me to steadfastness,
    to depend on you in the darkest of
night,
    surely able to sing of your faithfulness
to me.

Lord, in the constancy of the seasons and
in the course of the heavens,
    in the giving of pardon and peace, sure
    witness to your great faithfulness
    is seen, valued and taken to heart.

Lord, your faithfulness strengthens bright
hope in me for tomorrow;
    may my faith sow the seeds of faith in
    others, giving trust
    into the hearts of those whose pains
    and sorrows I share.

Thy hand hath provided – great is thy faithfulness, Lord, unto me!

Lord, may I follow in your footsteps, reck-
lessly giving away my faith,
    trusting mine shall remain and grow
    and not diminish in the giving;
    for I lose no light when my candle
    lights that of another.

Lord, graciously allow such freedom of
faith in the way that I am day by day,
    and in the sort of trust I show when
    meeting the needs of others,
    that your gift of faith may be accepted
    and treasured by them.   Amen.

WORKING WITH OTHERS

He who receives you receives me,
and he who receives me receives him who sent me.

Jesus (Matthew 10.40)

There was once a large institution serving many, many people in need. To make the whole thing work required considerable co-operation by a variety of professions and services. This was mostly organized in the usual, fairly bureaucratic way. Things generally worked together for good, but without feeling very stimulating.

There were, however, two areas of endeavour which were recognized as more specialized. The ambience of these two units felt quite different: well focused and highly motivated. They were in separate buildings from the rest, one not even on the same site. It was the teamwork that was distinctive. The senior professional, in each case with a particular charisma and personal authority, enabled teams from different professions and agencies to work closely and effectively together. Gifts and graces, skills and experiences were accepted openly. If it was the cleaner who had a special grandmotherly pastoral care for the teenagers then that was valued and used.

They felt good places to be but there were two sides to the story.
There was much sharing but it could be very challenging.

There was much that was radical but it could become threatening.

Life felt adventurous but could also feel 'on the edge' professionally.

The pace was exciting but could be relentless too.

There was close support but it could be confrontational.

There was strong loyalty but no room for passengers, who could feel uncomfortable.

Most of us are only too well aware of the two sides to working with others. Those of us who come from professions that traditionally worked as sole practitioners may be well aware of the advantages and the frustrations of both systems. Those who care mostly on their own at home would often be glad of more understanding and support day by day.

When we work together with others we know the whole is greater than the sum of the parts, even though the parts can be awkward or brilliant, square pegs or fit like a glove, dependable or weak links.

There is no perfect team, no perfect team member, and each of us is an imperfect candidate. When Jesus called the twelve to be apostles, and then seventy to be ministers of gospel power, he knew all this. Despite their faults, and the evident dangers, he sent them out in mini teams of two, to great effect. A pattern was set for corporate working, shared ministry and pastoral or clinical practice that we can respect today. The gospel teaches us that he promises us, through his Holy Spirit, wisdom and strength; he respects those decisions upon which we agree, and then put before him in intercession. Thus we may invite him always to be part of our team – or, should we say, he has invited us to be part of his team!

WORKING WITH OTHERS

There are lots of different kinds of nuts in the Lord's fruitcake.

Walter Hearn

Thank you, Lord, for giving me others to work with. I do appreciate it.

We are all strings in the concert of His joy.
Jakob Bohme
(1575–1624)

Thank you for putting teams together, and for the mutual respect we have for one another.
Help me with those few whose gifts I find it more difficult to discern.

Thank you especially for those who know what I find difficult and why.
Thank you for their understanding; thank you for giving them insight.
I know that some have gained that insight through their own particular problems, faithfully worked through.

Forgive me for being a little difficult at times.
Forgive me that there is that in me which some seem allergic to –
A nut allergy! – and I readily admit that I do have my little quirks.
If I am to be a nut, help me to be sweet, and not rancid, I pray.

Help us to gain insights from one another.
Help us not to consider ourselves as the first in the team.
How easily we do it!
Help us to serve one another in little ways, like making a cup of coffee.
And when grief comes, help us to uphold one another in love.

I lift to you these special people who give of themselves to care with me, Lord:
Please bless them, encourage them, give them your strength and your joy in all they do, in Jesus' name.

Amen.

If I cannot do great things, I can do small things in a great way.
James Freeman Clark (1810–88)

LISTENING

And a voice came out of the cloud, saying,
'This is my Son, my Chosen; listen to him.'

Luke 9.35

Listening is a key part of caring. It is not an easy option. Those most skilled in the practice tell of the awareness and alertness needed, of the proactive nature of what they do and the patience required, using counselling skills that enable a client to feel heard, understood and accepted.

For many of us tensions arise. It not just time. If the time allowed for appointments is ten minutes or less in a busy practice how can one hope to listen effectively? If there are practical things like exercises to be done, or it is in the middle of the drug round, or you have to listen to the heart beat – how can one hear the heart cry at any depth? Yet we know that to treat the whole person we need to hear both.

It is also so easy to jump ahead of the game – we have seen it all before, heard it often – experience tells us what is wrong, and what the best answer might be. We could so easily cut straight through all the verbiage, and offer the solution directly. But how will our parishioner, client, patient feel then: unheard, not understood, dissatisfied, asking if they have really met with their carer?

For the carer at home it may be the other way round. With all the time in the world, nothing much is ever shared, or only the same complaints and worries. There is the grief of hearing little of sense from the partner of many years, now suffering from Alzheimer's. A parent's heart sinks as she realizes, deep down, she may never hear more than grunts from the growing child who is dumb. All this does not mean there is no communication, but it is not the same. We grow to be well aware of body language and the meanings of little signals, the unspoken calls, the wordless messages that come from those whom the world may consider the least worthy.

When it is a struggle to listen, to whom are we listening? In the parable of the last judgement Jesus names people for whom listening is a major element of their care: the stranger, the sick, the imprisoned. Some of the most imprisoned in our society are those who carry a heavy burden of care at home. Ultimately, it is the Lord to whom we are called to listen. What a privilege! What a responsibility! How challenging is it to listen to him? Listening to him in other people may be our vocation. Let us remember we are also called to listen to him for ourselves.

While for the crowds in Galilee listening to Jesus seems to have been a captivating experience, for many of us it is a testing experience – more of a listening for Jesus. Will he speak to us, to me? How? How can I be sure it is him? We may be asking, where is God in all this? Has he got something to say to me? In the noisy turmoil of life, of our work, of our caring, how can I listen for the voice of God? In reflection we almost certainly shall be aware of new meanings and directions, understandings and insights. Remember that the Holy Spirit is expert in wordless messages. Through his prompting good counsel and divine wisdom come to those who wait.

LISTENING

Lord, my nature is not to listen. It's not my fault; it's how you made me!

No, my child, it is not how I made you.

But, Lord, I'm <u>good</u> at cutting through the verbiage and coming up with the solution! Why waste time?

People need to be heard. That's why I'm listening to you now. Or would you rather have the solution, in a nutshell, and stop wasting time?

Well, no, Lord; I guess we'll get to it once I know you understand how I feel . . .

Quite. You're learning! Actually, I do understand, completely – which, if I might say so gently, my child, is more than you do with you-know-who.

You don't mind if I just spill out all this stuff, then, Lord? Even if I did it for half an hour, without drawing breath, like you-know-who does with me?

No, I count it a joy that you want to fellowship with me. It's what I made you for. (She does draw breath, by the way.)

You mean you don't even want to make a little point to unravel the whole problem?

No. You'll get there. I might lead you beside still waters for a while, or show you a daisy close up, or lay on a thunderstorm, or light up a verse from my Word, or show you a great child of mine suffering-with-joy, or ask you a question which will lead you to the real answer if you think and pray it through; but I'm not going to short circuit the learning process. Why would I? Quickly learned lessons are quickly forgotten.

God has given one tongue but two ears that we may hear twice as much as we speak.
Anon.

Dear Lord, then help me to learn from you, and to listen better – to you, to others – and not to think that you have made me their oracle (or, indeed, yours – the very thought of it!).

Help me instead to listen patiently, to reflect back to them, and to lead them on in ways that help them to find their own solution; help me to lay aside my cleverness . . .

I will. I will, my beloved child. Just rest in me, and come and talk often – at any time, in any place; learn from me, and find rest for your soul.

Amen!

UNDERSTANDING

O Lord, you have searched me out and
known me,
You know my sitting down and my rising up;
You discern my thoughts from afar.
You mark out my journeys and my resting
place,
and are acquainted with all my ways.

Psalm 139.2–3

There are levels of understanding.

The basic level, when it comes to disease, is to recognize it for what it is; to put a diagnosis to it – a truthful diagnosis, insofar as we are able.

But to understand truly, we have to gain an understanding of the one afflicted, and perceive how the diagnosis, the condition, impacts upon them.

Only then can we truly be entering into the realm of care of the whole person.

Sometimes I think I understand everything; then I regain consciousness.
Ashleigh Brilliant

Understanding the entirety – the disease, the patient and the interplay between the two – is infinitely more demanding than the merely scientific approach. Here lies something of the art of medicine; the art of intervention not just with skill but with sensitivity, too.

A particular malady can mean profoundly different things to different people. One sufferer can simply regret that it has been visited upon them; another, because of a negative past experience of that condition, will be profoundly fearful. This is an example of the complex interplay between malady and sufferer.

Again, for some the personal or financial consequences of becoming well may be so adverse that they simply cannot become well. The malady has paradoxically benefited them either financially or through the attention and care it has earned them. Better to be ill than well.

Time with the sufferer and their family allows these interplays to come to light and be explored.

In truth, we need the deeper insights and gifts of the Holy Spirit as we walk with the diseased.

And we are reminded that we alone might not have everything necessary for the one for whom we care. That's alright. God made us to work in teams; we need one another.

UNDERSTANDING

O Lord, you have searched me out and known me;
you discern my thoughts from afar.
You . . . are acquainted with all my ways.

> Lord, it is a little disturbing to think you know me so
> well; there are parts of my story, I confess, that I would
> prefer to keep hidden.
> But I perceive in my heart that you care; it is for
> my own good that you know my depths, so your
> cleansing may cover all of my need.

For there is not a word on my tongue,
but you, O Lord, know it altogether.

> Lord, may you guide the words on my tongue when I
> seek to understand another person.
> Guide my listening and deepen my insight, I pray,
> that I may be led to greater appreciation.

. . . even darkness is no darkness with you;
the night is as clear as the day;
darkness and light to you are both alike.

> There are times, Lord, when I seem thick, missing the
> importance in symptoms or stories, when I am blind
> to meanings or feelings.
> Open my inner eyes and rouse my heart, I pray, throw
> your light before me to make it all clear.

I thank you, for I am fearfully and wonderfully made;
marvellous are your works, my soul knows well.

> Lord, I marvel at how wonderfully you have made
> us, yet I cannot interpret all the intricacies that make
> body, soul and spirit interact.
> So help me, Lord, to realize your creative love for
> each one who comes seeking good counsel and care;
> inspire in me, I pray, the gift of discernment.

How deep are your counsels to me, O God!
How great is the sum of them!

> Lord, I praise you for all that you have shown me, for
> all that I have realized by the nudging of your spirit.
> You alone have given me the empathy and insights
> that enable me to relate with understanding.

Search me out, O God and know my heart;
Try me and examine my thoughts.

> Enfold in your care, ever compassionate Lord, all
> whom I meet; may they feel heard, understood and
> treated with respect.
> May we share and hold together in trust what we grasp
> by the work of your Spirit.
> Pray let the depth of your wisdom guide us, each and
> all, into your eternal wholeness.

. . . and lead me in the way everlasting. Amen.
(Quotations are from Psalm 139)

PATIENCE

*The fruit of the Spirit is love, joy, peace,
patience,
kindness, goodness, faithfulness, self-control.*

Galatians 5.22

Occasionally I am brought to recognize that I need patience – more patience than I have.

Sadly, the most needy can tax my patience most – often because their need is not just physical, but emotional and spiritual – and those needs can be untidy and difficult to address.

Dear God, please grant me patience. And I want it now.
Anon.

So, when we are tired and tested, and presented with seemingly impossible situations, what can we do?

Yes, pray for patience, and repent of impatience – that is vital.

But it may be that things need not be quite so impossibly complex at all; it may be that there is a practical solution to much of the difficulty; so to pray for problem-solving skills, and the winsomeness to present a solution in an acceptable way, might be helpful too.

Never cut what you can untie.
Joseph Joubert
(1754–1824)

It may be that our expectations don't match those of the one for whom we care: we need to pray for insight and understanding.

It may be that we aren't the right people to provide the input on this occasion; do we need to involve a counsellor? – or a pastor? Or just someone with a little more time to listen – someone outside the situation, perhaps? Our inclination is to take the whole load; but are we taking on too much? We might thereby be blocking input from the very person needed.

Patience is the ability to put up with people you'd like to put down.
Ulrike Ruffert

We might be taking on too much . . . surely better to recognize the fact and get someone else involved than yielding to impatience.

So, faced with feelings of impatience, whether with patient, sick relative, client or parishioner, we need to take time to consider: is this my lack, or are there other issues to consider? The question needs to be asked.

Moreover, we need to know where to turn if things don't improve. Counsellors are good at recognizing when they need help; nurses, doctors and ministers tend to be less so, on the whole. But for us all, it is at times important to hear the detached perspective of a wise colleague or friend who knows what it is to be led of the Spirit; who will not just sympathize but reflect; even challenge, where necessary.

Take rest! A field that has rested gives a bountiful crop.
Ovid (43BC–17AD)

And finally, we all need to holiday at times: a regular Sabbath (or equivalent), and a longer break at regular intervals. That is good for everyone.

PATIENCE

Now the God of patience and consolation
grant you to be likeminded one to another according to
Christ Jesus:
That ye may with one mind and one mouth glorify God,
even the Father of our Lord Jesus Christ.

Romans 15.5 (AV)

Fatherly God, I am praying while mulling over deep matters;
I am amazed at the endless patience and kindness you have
for people like me. How wonderful you are!

> I realize how slow I have been to follow your word,
> when you had so often made everything plain.

> Foolishly I have leapt off at a tangent, I confess:
> leaving your way, when it was clear before me.

Lord, have mercy; Christ, have mercy; Lord, have mercy.

Lord Jesus Christ, I thank you for your great patience with
me;
You seem always ready to wait and to forgive, to dust me
down and set me going again.

> I have to confess my frustrations show quickly.
> You know I have never suffered fools gladly.

> I realize there is so much I should learn from you:
> All about the nature of patience and long-suffering.

Lord, have mercy; Christ, have mercy; Lord, have mercy.

O Spirit of the living God, I thank you for the gifts you give, like peace, humility and self-control that prepare me for the gift of patience.

> Plant such fruits of your Spirit in my soul, I pray, and by your tender nurture grow them strong.

> With grace may I endure delay and waste of effort; and with forbearance help those who irritate.

Lord, have mercy; Christ, have mercy; Lord, have mercy.

O Trinity of patient love, I commend to you in my prayer all situations or folk who try my patience: let your long-suffering kindness greet them.

> I pray that if it is one I love, with whom I lack stamina, calm my tone, relax their mood, let peace return.
> Help us rid ourselves of everything that gets in the way, and run with patience the race that lies before us.

Praise God from whom all mercies flow;
praise him all creatures here below,
praise him above, ye heavenly host;
praise Father, Son and Holy Ghost. Amen.

PERSEVERANCE

*Therefore, my beloved, be steadfast,
immoveable, always excelling in the work of
the Lord, because you know that in the Lord
your labour is not in vain.*

1 Corinthians 15.58

*Great works are
performed not by
strength but by
perseverance.*
Samuel Johnson

On a bright summer's day, when we are young, fit and eager, how gladly and readily can we make promises that carry awesome responsibilities. 'I take you . . . to have and to hold . . . for better, for worse . . . in sickness and in health; to love and to cherish; till death . . .' Till when? An awful lot can happen before death. Some of it can be chronic disease or disability. Having and holding may have serious consequences.

*Who would true
valour see, let him
come hither;
One here will
constant be,
come wind come
weather;
There's no
discouragement
shall make him
once relent
His first avowed
intent to be a
pilgrim.*
John Bunyan

Responsibility for continuing care can arise in all of the close family relationships, and will usually imply long-term dedication. We can have no idea how long we shall be taking the strain of bearing the burden of a carer; nor little idea of how things may deteriorate, nor of the time needed each day, nor of the tedious weight of the work.

What sort of perseverance do we need? What will keep us steadfast, constantly ready to care and to serve through thick and thin, through fire and water? What

I can plod. I can persevere in any definite pursuit. To this I owe everything.
William Carey

will help us keep right on to the end of the road? We can readily see some qualities that will be very valuable, for example: inner or outer strength; resolute demeanour; sense of humour; emotional balance; a persistent attitude; the ability to plod; and so forth.

Clearly the will is important; the willingness to ask for help, again and again, and not be fobbed off. It sounds like obstinacy, but there is a difference. Henry Ward Beecher, the American preacher and journalist, put it like this: 'The difference between perseverance and obstinacy is, that one comes from a strong will, and the other from a strong won't.' There will be arduous times for all of us, whether caring at home, or in the clinical or pastoral settings. We will need to be diligent and vigorous in meeting recurring difficulties.

Lord God, when you call your servants to endeavour any great matter, grant us also to know that it is not the beginning, but the continuing of the same, until it be thoroughly finished, which yields the true glory; through him who, for the finishing of your work, laid down his life for us, our Redeemer, Jesus Christ. Amen.
Sir Francis Drake

Above all what we will need is grace – the help of Christ's unwearying constancy – to enable us to be gracious and forbearing, whatever has been messed up yet again. Then we will be well on the way to repeat the answer made long years before to the question, 'Will you love, comfort, honour and protect her/him, in sickness and in health'; With the help of God, one said, 'I will.' Surely it is God's will that you and I are enabled to keep our word.

PERSEVERANCE

*Teach us, good Lord, to serve you as you
deserve; to give and not to count the cost;
to fight and not to heed the wounds; to toil
and not to seek for rest; to labour and not to
ask for any reward save that of knowing we
do your will; through Jesus Christ our Lord.
Amen.*

St Ignatius Loyola

I never knew it would be like this.

Not that I would have done anything differently; but I had not taken on board the degree of responsibility; how much I would have to put aside what I want in order to care properly.

I need to see. Lord, I need to see the eternal significance of this.

I am not good at persevering; please help me by showing me how you see things.

Our Lord does not care so much for the importance of our works as for the love with which they are done.

St Teresa of Avila

I see things through the eye of love. Follow love and you will not go far wrong. Love is patient, love is kind, love does not envy, love is not puffed up, nor rude, nor self-seeking, is not easily provoked, thinks no evil and rejoices in the truth. Love bears all things, believes all things, hopes all things, endures all things. Follow love.

Even love changes! There was a time when love was as much about getting as giving – it was a mutual thing . . .

It still is. But the rewards are deeper, stronger and more enduring. This love of which I speak is the laying-down-your-life sort; it carries great rewards, though it looks sombre and forbidding. The reward only comes when the resentment is overcome, when you have given up all your hopes and dreams for the sake of love. Then you find that I am with you, for I know this kind of love so very well. It is agape love. And where I find it, I make my home, assuming I am welcomed.

You are welcomed! How can I cope without you? Teach me, comfort me, transform me, for I am needy and vulnerable; I could so easily give up . . .

Do you want to?

No, I really don't. I want to succeed in loving truly – I want to do your will, my Lord and my God . . .

Not your will, but mine? Then we'll share the fellowship of agape, of self-sacrificial love, and you will know me present with you, and I shall transform and strengthen you. I shall never leave you, nor forsake you . . .

AWKWARDNESS

Jesus knew their thoughts . . .

Matthew 12.25

*Never argue with
another: remember
he too has a right
to his own stupid
opinion.*
Anon.

At times, people we care for are just plain awkward! Others just *seem* awkward because they are simply inept with words. It is for us to discern the difference, and win the awkward in speech by interpreting their words generously, reacting graciously.

Others are impossibly verbose; they simply can't prioritize their thinking and tell their story in chronological sequence. Such people can be helped. One might say, for example, 'Good morning, it's good to see you. Well, we have a full fifteen minutes. Tell me the *most* important thing on your mind, so at least we'll have covered *that* today.'

What of those who really are very demanding, or difficult, or hostile? We need to be clear in our minds what is a reasonable expectation, and what is unreasonable. And then we need gently to clarify that to them. Perhaps we need to recognize that Jesus had his limits; so do we.

And for those of us who are professional carers – what about the litigious? The one who tells you he's taken legal action against the consultant, the counsellor and others – and thereby puts you on your back foot? Many of us incline to avoid confrontation, but perhaps a clear statement that the therapeutic relationship is founded on trust both ways, with the expressed hope that this will be possible, may not go amiss.

Anger is quieted by a gentle word just as fire is quenched by water.
Jean Pierre Camus
(1584–1652)

Jesus was not available at the drop of a hat. Neither can we be.

Jesus did not persevere beyond measure with those who would not heed him: he spoke truth and left them to digest it. So may we, albeit always aware of our fallibility.

Jesus was wise in his dealings with those who in some way sought his harm. So should we be.

But Jesus also succeeded in recognizing a Nicodemus out of the Pharisees: he read the spirit of the person. So must we.

For out of the abundance of the heart the mouth speaks.
Luke 6.45b

And, though he burned against institutional injustice and the corruption of the Word of God, he ran on love. Even in the midst of our limitations and finite energy, we too must run on love.

It is perhaps a question of having the same attitude as Jesus, who recognized the good heart and responded graciously, while yet neither giving of himself to those without ears to hear, nor surrendering himself into the hands of those who sought his harm – until the right time came.

And Jesus, looking at him, loved him . . .
Mark 10.21

AWKWARDNESS

*Because you have made the Lord your refuge
and the Most High your stronghold,
there shall no evil happen to you,
neither shall any plague come near your tent.*

Psalm 91.9, 10

O Lord my God, Most High, Almighty, full of compassion and mercy and love, I rejoice in your provision for our protection, for your holy angels give us our security.

*For he shall give
his angels charge
over you,
to keep you in all
your ways.
They shall bear
you in their hands,
lest you dash your
foot against a
stone.*
Psalm 91.11, 12

O Lord my God, you are our refuge and our hiding place. I praise you that despite all the snares, and the sneaky temptations, we may feel guarded against awkward traps; you, Lord, are the one who keeps us safe.

*Keep me as the
apple of your eye;
hide me under the
shadow of your
wings.*
Psalm 17.8

But, O my Lord, I do not really want to be hidden away from those who are in my care, nor from their awkwardness, for they are often unable to come with dignity.

My Lord, I need your grace, your compassion, your wisdom and good counsel, that I may see each clumsy one with your insight, and react with your kind of treatment.

I pray you, O Lord, for steadfast love so I

may reach out to the hearts and souls of those I find awkward. Use me I pray to respond with kindness and clarity, to allay their fears with sympathy and understanding.

I think of those who cannot help their genetic inheritance; in Galilee and Judah you met each one just as she or he was. Your mercy is even for the bully: have pity on him. Those with learning difficulties can receive you gladly.

You, Lord, are patient and reassuring to the worried well; you understand how anxiety can cripple. Have mercy on attention seekers in their desperation to find dependable love and value; pray assist me to respond with the right kind of welcome.

Your heart, O Lord, still reaches out to those who rejected you, to all who feel they need to fight for their right to receive care. Your wisdom meets the one whose question is hostile. Your truth was, and is, always just to the mind of the lawyer.

Save, Lord, all those of us who need saving from ourselves; may our ears and hearts be open and ready for you. Whatever we are like, you have already met people like us and given the hope of healing, wholeness and salvation.

FOR THE LEAST OF THESE . . .

*I'm telling the solemn truth: whenever you
did one of these things to someone overlooked
or ignored, that was me – you did it to me.*

Jesus (Matthew 25.40)

This text comes from Jesus' story about the judgement at his second coming. The ones who will be blessed are those who met the King's needs; the test of which would be in how one had treated the most needy people. Many of us have volunteered to care for such as these; it is only later we find ourselves face to face with those whom we judge the least worthy. It is very challenging.

It is certainly very difficult to see Christ in many people. I have to ask myself: on whom do I look down? From whom do I recoil? For example, I find it enormously difficult to see Christ in someone who has utterly degraded him or herself. Most of us could probably make a list. How on earth can I see Christ in these?

Bless those who curse you, pray for those who abuse you.
Jesus (Luke 6.28)

Perhaps that is the point; you can't see him in them. They might repel us, whereas we expect Christ to attract us. Our vocation is to serve their needs as if we did see Christ in them, impossible though it might be to envisage him. It is a matter of the will – choosing to serve those to whom we are not naturally attracted. God can use your clinical, reasoned detachment – he asks for your commitment and determination.

The question becomes: what do I have to overcome in myself? Am I one who recoils from whining complaints, or fears contagion of any sort, or who is turned off by manipulations and attention-seeking behaviour? Unless I am in denial, I will have to address my revulsion, my selfishness, or my feeling of resentment at being put on the spot by a beggar – and that includes the unsolicited appeals that drop through my letter box.

But you may be someone who has a natural compassion for those in great need. The world is a better place for people blessed with such a gift. Thankfully we recall Mother Teresa and her community; or Jean Vanier and L'arche, though we note in the writings of Henri Nouwen that committing oneself to this life can be most testing. God the ever merciful can make good use of your gifting, your involvement and your love. Yet the spontaneity of your response to the beggar may still need to be tempered by discretion, as you ask yourself: what is really the best for her or him?

FOR THE LEAST OF THESE . . .

> *Look! A leper is approaching. He kneels*
> *before Jesus, worshipping.*
> *'Sir', the leper pleads, 'if you want to, you can*
> *heal me.'*
> *Jesus touches the man. 'I want to,' he says, 'be*
> *healed.'*
>
> Matthew 8.2, 3 (Living Bible)

Lord, you touched the lepers . . . and I sometimes find it difficult to cope with the merely awkward.

(*And* the forgetful who repeat themselves, *and* those who – well, those with all sorts of problems.)

Help me to overcome all the feelings I know are negative.

When I look at these, these who arouse such negative thoughts in me, I realize that I might be like them in such a very short time, and then I think those who care for me might think the same things that I'm thinking now; and I don't know how I could cope with that . . .

Lord, help me to see just a little of you in each one I care for; help me to put myself in their shoes, and ask whether, honestly, I'd do any better than they're doing.

How I hope I would! How I hope I'd be bright, and courteous, and grateful, and humorous!

But in truth I'm afraid that I'll be crabby, short-tempered, ungrateful – and then try and put it all right in a few words. I'd lurch from grotty to great in a moment; but most of the time I'd be grotty.

Hear me, Lord; I'm crying out to you! – and I'm not doing too well, in case you hadn't noticed . . . Let me start again; give me grace to say how sorry I am that I'm sometimes short, sometimes resentful, sometimes less caring than I would have believed possible in a carer. Help me to walk in the shoes of the one I care for, for just a little while – not to actually be ill, you understand, but to be able to comprehend better where they're coming from.

I thought one was supposed to get more saintly as one grows older. One is? And this is the way you're teaching me?

I'd rather have a temperament transplant! – not possible? Then I know I need to change. So do what's needed, Lord. Show me what I need to see in order to make that change.

And I shall worship you as I see you working this rough old clay that's me into something that's a bit more like you.

We do pray for mercy; and that same prayer doth teach us all to render the deed of mercy.
William Shakespeare
(1564–1616)

NOTHING
WE CAN DO

Surely he has born our griefs, and carried our sorrows.

Isaiah 53.4 (RSV)

There comes a day when the tough diagnosis has to be shared. We know we have reached the limits of our professional resources. How do we share such bad news? How do we feel about giving what may sound like a death sentence? What does it do to us, and how do we cope?

Walking the tightrope of perceptions, feeling our patient's shock on the one hand and on the other hand needing to retain our dispassionate role we are torn. With experience we learn ways of handling the consultation, yet always it will be new and personal. Even as hearts sink at the bleak prospect, we see the disbelief and baffled look in the eyes of the other; or is it the nod of one who had suspected?

Then there are the temptations: wrap the news up carefully with empty euphemisms; or be so blunt there can be no mistake. For me it came in the out-patients department: she looked me in the eyes and shocked me with the sentence, 'There is no cure.' But I went home revived with a treatment plan that was to bring rapid and amazing alleviation of symptoms. Sacramental ministry also played its part. Yet the threat remains.

Bad enough as such moments are for the professional, of whatever calling, it is so much more desperate for those of us who care for family, when we realize we must finally admit, 'There is nothing more I can do for you.' The limit has been reached, for whatever reason. Here there is no professionalism behind which to hide. One only had oneself: one's love, devotion and commitment to offer – no techniques, treatments or special skills.

Might it even mean we can no longer live together in our own home? Having done our best, it can feel as if we are letting down and failing the one for whom we have given so much. This is a deeply disappointing and frustrating moment, grievous to contemplate. But is there really 'nothing we can do'? Practical help to cope with tough reality is possible.

We can always be of one heart, grieve together, stay alongside come what may; even if we need to refer. To feel one has nothing to offer is not a matter of failing or guilt; it is a sharing of human vulnerability. When I as a carer am open about my limitations, the one for whom I care can appreciate that. If we can together follow that path where nearly nothing is possible, in the clinical sense, we may find mutual strength in the emotional and spiritual areas.

This does not take away the loss or frustration; but it does allow us to take hold of it and live it out in relationship; even with one, far better equipped than we, who has grieved before us. Thinking of the rich young man, some of the Pharisees, the city of Jerusalem and Judas Iscariot, how much did Christ weep for, and on behalf of, those for whom there seemed to be nothing he could do?

NOTHING WE CAN DO . . .

Dear Lord, this is so difficult – please help me . . .

I struggle both with my own feelings, and with finding something positive to say – I am oppressed by the negative.

There is a haunted look within the eyes of the one for whom I am caring; 'the game's up', they say, and challenge me to say differently. And I hunt for that positive way of putting things.

*We hope vaguely
But dread
precisely.*
Paul Valéry
(1871–1945)

'Where there's life there's hope' – ? Yes, but not a lot. 'Look on the bright side' – ? What bright side?

Deliver me, O Lord! Help me!

Pilgrimages have beginnings and endings, but they are always with purpose, and nothing that happens is random; all is born of my love. Tune in to my love; feel it resting over you both, all the more as the trials come. I will strengthen, if you will lean on me . . .

Lord, this whole problem of mortality, and of sickness, is unutterably depressing; even a step forward will inevitably be

*O Lord, my heart
is not lifted up, my
eyes are not raised
too high. I will not
occupy myself with
things too great
and too marvellous
for me. But I
have calmed and
quieted my soul,
like a child quieted
at its mother's
breast; like a child
that is quieted
is my soul. Oh
Israel! Hope in the
Lord! – from this
time forth and for
ever more!*
From Psalm 131

*Trust involves
letting go and
knowing that God
will catch you.*
James Dobson
(1936–)

swallowed up in a step back before so very
long . . .

*I know. It is the curse you inherit; but be of
good cheer. I have overcome it! And I invite
you to join the celebration of love in my kingdom – soon . . . just trust me, follow me, love
with my love . . .*

And how do I do that? In this awful situation, where there seems nothing that can
be done – how do I care?

*You take too much upon yourself. You look for
the philosophical answer, the theological solution, and you assume guilt if you can't find
it. Be a child! Enough that I know all things;
I will reveal to you what you need to know – at
the right time. Let go of the need to know all
the answers. The time of knowing will come.
Right now, it's the time for trusting. You want
to know how to care? 'Do unto others as you
would have them do unto you.' Love, laugh
and pray; the one you care for is the one I care
for too. Relax in my love! – and spread my
joy.*

No more than that? I just rest in you,
quieten my soul in your love, and love as
you have loved me? Help me, then, Lord,
to keep focused on you and not on the
questions . . .

NEARLY NOTHING
TO OFFER

In the tender compassion of our God the dawn from
on high shall break upon us,
to shine on those who dwell in darkness and the
shadow of death,
and to guide our feet into the way of peace.

Luke 1.78, 79 (*Common Worship*)

There are days when we, either as professionals or carers at home, are at our limits with virtually nothing helpful to offer. Easily we can feel inadequate and impotent, as carers, or in ourselves. The reactions we meet may deepen these feelings. Suppose your client, patient, parishioner, or loved one would actively welcome a terminal prognosis. What does that do to you? A true parable can illustrate some of the issues with which we wrestle.

'Gwen' suffered under the curse of a serious psychotic diagnosis. Twenty-five years or so ago, she lived long term in a ward in the old county 'Asylum', renamed 'Hospital'. She was on heavy medication; a bag lady stalking the interminable corridors. At least she had shelter, warmth, three meals a day, and was accepted just for who she was, at her ports of call.

The Hospital Library was her place. Rather than sit around all day patients were organised to work, or therapy or diversion. As an Oxford graduate Gwen had much to offer in the library.

But there were many days when Gwen just needed to crash out. She would come to the church, put cushions on the floor and sleep in her own mini-asylum.

In church was, though, where she could express her torment. At the altar rail as she lifted her hand she would look me in the eye and say, 'I pray only to die.' Remembering the laments of the Psalmist, there was no way I could condemn that prayer, or refuse Communion. As her prayer reached up, so I reached down with the sign of the broken body deliberately given through death for her; given to set her free from her torments; given too to strengthen all those of us who suffered her prayer with nearly nothing to offer.

So finally, on Boxing day Gwen took refuge in the loo with one of her plastic bags and answered her own prayer.

At her funeral, where she lay resting for the last time in an earthly house of God I was surprised how many were present. No family, but staff, volunteers, patients: despite all, could we be called 'family and friends'? It seemed as though when we had nearly nothing to offer she had been offering something to us. She had called us to share, not just compassion, but common human helplessness. So we commended her to the God who had reached out to her prayer and prepared a perfect asylum for her in a better place.

There was nearly nothing more to do, except comfort each other; and let the realization dawn upon us that in the moment when Christ, his body broken on the Cross, had nearly nothing he could do, he had in fact offered all he could and done everything that was actually needed. Perhaps God could, would and did accept the nearly nothing we had offered.

NEARLY NOTHING
TO OFFER

I want to give what is necessary, Lord.

I want to have answers. Yet you seem not
to want to let me.

*No. I am the way, the truth and the life. You
seem to want to usurp that.*

No, I don't! I just hate feeling so helpless.
There seems nothing I can do. Or is there?

*Of course there is! You are already caring.
Now ask yourself; what do you want from me?
For yourself? For the one for whom you care?*

What do I want for me? That has something to do with it? O, Lord, thou knowest;
I want peace, patience, endurance, love,
wisdom . . .

Granted.

WHAT? Granted? What do you mean?
How do I get hold of them?

*Through one prayer at a time, my child. Don't
be upset! You need petrol for the car; you don't
get a year's supply at one go – do you? The tank
isn't big enough. And I've got news for you:
nor is your peace-patience-love-endurance-
wisdom tank! But here is my credit card.
When you need these things, ask my Father*

*Hitherto you have
asked nothing in
my name. Ask,
and you will
receive, that your
joy may be full!*
John 16.24

and show him this. Yes; it's a cross. It's good for salvation, too. Use it – as soon as you're running low.

I ran out months ago. I need the rescue service!

Most people do. All my resources, any time – and you run out! Why not keep the tank half full at least? You're behaving like a man!! – waiting 'til the little red light flashes! Don't. Come often; and have a chat while you're at it. I love to see you; I love your love, your fellowship. I will warm you, dry your tears, reassure you and fill your tank. If you run out, you have a little extra walk, a few more tears, a lot more anxiety . . .

Human fellowship can go to great lengths, but not all the way. Fellowship with God can go to all lengths.
Oswald Chambers
(1874–1917)

I get the point. But what about the one I care for? What about her? Will you talk to her, too? And give her all she needs for the journey ahead? Yes, I am hearing you. You will. And I don't have to be God. OK. All I have to do is care, right? Well, I do!! Oh, Lord, joy is filling my heart . . . fill my tank and let me go; I'm ready! And thank you, Lord, so very much. I worship you. You have the words of eternal life, and they are like honey in my mouth . . .

Yes. Don't forget my great love for the one you care for so faithfully. There is one more thing you can do . . . like you, she puts off coming to me. Gently remind her that I'm always waiting for her. Offer to come with her . . . For my love overflows for you both.

THE CROSS

*Most assuredly, I say to you, when you
[Simon] were younger, you girded yourself
and walked where you wished; but when you
are old, you will stretch out your hands, and
another will gird you and carry you where you
do not wish to go.*

John 21.18

None of us want to suffer; none of us want
to witness suffering.

But suffering is a part of our lot. Few of us
avoid it.

Thankfully, we can alleviate it – and that is
the desire of every carer.

Yet it remains, and inevitably we as carers
take a portion of the suffering of the one
for whom we care. That can't be avoided,
except by not caring.

Is it possible that suffering can be trans-
formed in some way?

Perhaps it depends on our frame of refer-
ence.

When Jesus spoke about 'carrying our
cross', referring to the possibility of suffering, he wasn't referring to *all* suffering.

People suffer: not all of it is to do with
bearing a cross.

The cross relates to that suffering which is
borne for Christ, because we are his.

On this basis, most of the world's suffering has little to do with the Cross save as a figure of speech.

Yet the ones who love Jesus live for him, and die for him: they make him their reason for living, and accept suffering at his hands, knowing that he works to produce fruit out of it.

That is the Cross.

Approaching suffering in this way requires courage.

Of course we alleviate suffering every way we can, cure with compassion when we have the means, and pray anyway.

But suffering remains a mystery. Can we as carers allow it to remain so? – by saying, 'I don't understand why this has to happen, but I'm here and standing by you: we'll walk together with Jesus.'

He understands the Cross fully; we do not. We must let him lead us and comfort us, and strengthen us, and change us, whether we are sufferer or carer.

And we must pray for the increasing reality of living, loving, suffering, laughing – whatever – all for him, our 'all in all'.

Carry the cross patiently and with perfect submission and in the end it shall carry you.
Thomas à Kempis
(c. 1380–1471)

THE CROSS

Jesus cried out with a loud voice, 'Eloi, Eloi, lema sabachthani'
which means, 'My God, my God, why have you forsaken me?'

Mark 15.34

In the silence of Good Friday I compose this prayer.
Lord Jesus Christ, my friend, my saviour,
today we have heard you pierce that dark hour
with your cry of desperation and abandonment.

Following the way of your Cross in our worship
has been utterly harrowing, as it always is.
Feeling the deep, deep sorrow of your mother
has literally brought tears to the eyes.

Your Cross, dear Jesus, so heavy, so rugged
on the wall of our church looked just too heavy.
Even for you it was too much – it got you down.
You needed help; to save us by the Cross you needed help.

As we prayed, this very day, dear Jesus, we were aware
there are many who are carrying their cross.
Some have denied themselves to take it up;
far more feel it thrust hard upon them.

Some cry out, desperate as you have been;
some fall under the weight, just as you crashed down.
Raise them up, Lord – relieve their pains, Lord.
Reach out, Lord, we pray, as you did to the dying thief.

How do you reach out, Lord? I am wondering.
I recall Simon, from Cyrene, and feel impelled to ask,
'Do you mean me to be a Simon?' To help someone,
to help carry the cross for those I love, I serve?

Dear Lord and Saviour, as I take up a cross with another
grant me your grace to do it in such a willing manner
he or she may feel true support, sharing and sympathy
so that they know it is really you, Jesus, sharing their cross.

Thus I bring to you the cross-bearers I know, or love;
all the ones who are mocked, scorned or abused.
I also bring people betrayed, denied or let down by friends,
all who are tortured, unjustly accused or convicted.

Give your strength and courage, dear Lord, to all those
who falteringly climb up to Calvary's cruel blows:
to pain, anguish of mind, dereliction of spirit.
Pray let all who reach their skull-shaped hill today
come to be with you, Jesus, in paradise.

We adore you, O Christ and we bless you;
by your holy Cross, you have redeemed the world.

THE GATES OF HEAVEN

Precious in his sight is the death of his saints . . .

Psalm 116.15

Caring for those we know to be terminally ill carries great challenges.

Everyone responds to the reality of their impending death in different ways.

Our caring may embrace many needs: from comforting the frightened, to reviewing the sufferer's life with them, to speaking with relatives, to the practical elements of care and symptom control, to prayer.

The keys to effective terminal care are respect, a difficult balance of seriousness and humour, and an acute awareness of the whole person we care for – spirit, soul and body.

Respect is love in plain clothes.
Frankie Byrne

But respect is the absolute foundation to all caring; no one feels cared for if not respected.

Seriousness says – 'I take you seriously, and you can say whatever you want; I won't make light of it.'

Laughter says – 'We can share fun in the most unexpected places; let's do so – as long as you want.' People feel better for humour, and, paradoxically, it enables deep conversation. It is a foil for over-intensity.

The physical environment is important, as is music known and loved, favourite scriptures and words of comfort, and the right people. All bring solace and comfort.

So he passed over, and all the trumpets sounded for him on the other side.
John Bunyan
(1628–88)

And awareness of the one cared for in totality means we can move from the physical to the emotional, to the intellectual, to the spiritual as the need arises.

Overarching all is the mystery of living and dying. No one who has accompanied someone to heaven's gates can fail to be aware of mystery, of changing state, of vacating of the body; it is a time of emotion and wonder.

But it can also be deeply upsetting, and we as carers need our own support, to debrief what we have felt, that our own grieving might be healthy.

Here is challenge, but as we love and care God will be with us.

THE GATES OF
HEAVEN

Jesus, like a mother you gather your people to you . . .
You comfort us in sorrow, you bind up our wounds,
in sickness you nurse us . . .
by your dying we are born to new life . . .

St Anselm

Jesus: Like a tender nurse, ever watchful and caring
you are full of compassion and mercy and love.
You learned so much from your holy mother
hearing her tell of the flight to Egypt, in fear of death;
her anguish over the death of the Holy Innocents
while you and she and Joseph were saved.

Jesus: With her you suffered the loss of faithful Joseph.
Perhaps you spoke with her to share comfort,
for both to be ready for that day the Cross tore you
apart.
It means much that you knew earthly sorrows and
distress.
You shared the grief and fear that foreshadows
death,
wept at the grave of a friend, and yet gave new life.

Jesus: Let love enfold all who now approach heaven's
gates.
Become real to the very young, and the innocent,
the very old or quite oblivious,

the deeply fearful, and all in denial,
the unprepared, and those who wait ready for the
   day,
those who know you well, or only in the passing.
Let your presence calm fears and give peace within;
may souls be made ready to greet your final call.

Jesus: You recognize the families, the friends along that
      road;
reach out to them in their bewilderment and grief,
understanding any anger and moments of guilt,
to bring your consolations and soothing relief.
Go with those who return alone from a bedside visit,
pray relieve the emptiness of the near silent home.

Jesus: I pray you for us who are called to care in your name:
you know what we go through as we try to cope.
Pray be at our side in the midst of trauma,
in moments of storytelling, relief or humour;
in the quiet times, prayer times, end time.
We too share the shocks, the sadness, the tears.
Pray grant us the reassurance of your consoling
   hand.

Jesus: Bless us and keep us all;
guard our bodies, save our souls
and bring us safe to that heavenly country,
our eternal home, where you
with the Father and the Holy Spirit reign,
one God for ever and ever. Amen.

UNDER PRESSURE

Jesus tells us his yoke is easy, his burden light; and as we take it up we will find rest for our souls (from Matthew 11.29, 30).

Then whose burdens are we carrying? – these that threaten to overwhelm us?

Thankfully, we know that we are not being promised freedom from pressures by Jesus' words, for the very disciples he addressed were soon to discover the ultimate pressures of persecution and martyrdom.

Thankfully? Yes; because otherwise *our* pressures, *our* trials would seem to be sin, in the light of Jesus' words.

In truth, he knows our pressures. He knows our limitations, too.

And he says 'Come unto me, you who labour and are heavy laden, and I will give you rest. Take my yoke upon you and learn from me, for I am gentle and lowly in heart, and you shall find rest for your souls' (Matthew 11.28–29).

Let's think about it. Where's the rest? It's for our souls – the innermost identity we possess. Interestingly, not necessarily for our bodies. And how do we get it? We take the yoke of Jesus, which is to learn his ways – which are gentleness and lowliness of heart.

The rest for our souls is not the result of moving from activity to inactivity; it is the result of an inner change of attitude.

No burden is too heavy when it is carried with love.
Anon.

It's an 'attitude check' we need.

Are we mirroring the gentleness of Jesus?

Are we lowly in heart? – not puffed up, not 'too good for this'; but lowly, and willing to be a servant, like Jesus?

It is in facing these things robustly and honestly that we will progress.

It is in talking to Jesus on the way, too, for caring *is* difficult, and hard work.

Collapse in the Christian life is seldom a blow-out; it is usually a slow leak.
Paul E. Little

And as our hearts mirror him in all gentleness and lowliness of heart, so our peace comes to us all over again.

And as we recognize that he *knows* where we are, he *knows* the trials we face, and he *knows* our future, so we find our purpose in his path for us. And all is well.

Every day laid down, every freedom forfeited, is known to God.

And he is the rewarder of all selflessness, all devotion, all love, and he gives his rewards both in this life and in eternity.

UNDER PRESSURE

*'Come to me, all you that are weary and are carrying heavy
burdens, and I will give you rest.'*
Jesus (Matthew 11.28–30)

Lord Jesus: Thank you for that invitation to come to you.
It is comforting just to hear your voice.
I am so weary – I do need the rest you offer.
The burden of it all seems so heavy,
and the days are so pressurized.
I am not good at finding a quiet spot in which to hide.

As I listen again to your words, Lord,
I realize it is not an invitation;
it is your command that I come to you for rest.
To come to you is a matter of obedience, of discipleship,
for you have my best interests in hand already.

Why do I find it so difficult to come to you, to turn to you?
I have to confess, Lord, that though you are my friend
it is often nearly the last thing I would do on my own.
But now I am here, pray help me let go of everything;
I think I need to just go flop, with you dear Lord.

*'Take my yoke upon you, and learn from me; for I am gentle
and humble in heart, and you will find rest for your souls.'*

Lord Jesus: I hear in this another command.
I must confess reluctance, diffidence,

about picking up any new burden;
At first glimpse this yoke looked rather like a cross,
though now I can feel how light it is.

I am amazed: you, the Lord of all power and might,
sovereign over all, judge of all souls,
are so very gentle alongside me now,
I am instantly at ease, your presence is so natural;
you set me free to be just the person I'm meant to be.

'For my yoke is easy, and my burden is light.'

Lord Jesus: you are making something wonderful happen.
I confess I doubted about what your yoke would do.
I thought it would weigh me down.
In reality it bears me up: Lord, how can I explain it?

It is as if the tide was coming in,
threatening to flood over me, swamp me,
and I feared I would lose my footing.
But your yoke is so carefully crafted and light it lifts me:
I float free – as if safely carried in your arms.

Lord Jesus, now I think no longer just of me.
For your love's sake, let those for whom I care
hear what is this marvel you can do.
I lift each one, especially the one nearest to me,
to find in you their rest, comfort and wholeness.

Lord Jesus, all praise and glory be to you for these great
mercies. Amen.

ISOLATED

*The hour is coming, indeed it has come,
when you will be scattered, everyone to his
home, and will leave me alone; yet I am not
alone, for the Father is with me.*

Jesus (John 16.32)

This is being written during 'Children in
need' week. Each day the local television
station has featured a charitable work
helping children. Today the cameras visited a project that brought together children who are 'carers' at home – they were
having a 'jam' session: lots of noise, lots of
fun, lots of release.

The interviews were touching: both the
matter-of-fact determination of children
bearing burdens of care, who did not
look old enough to be as far as secondary
school; the frustration and the gratitude of
a mother too chronically sick to do more
than the least of household chores. But
the key word was isolation – staying in to
care when one's peers were able to go out
and socialize. Thank God someone has
thought to include these hidden carers.

There comes a moment when any of us can
feel isolated in our caring work. For many

Pray that your loneliness may spur you into finding something to live for, great enough to die for.
Dag Hammarskjöld

at home it will be when we are physically on our own, with little support or no one with whom to talk over the situation.

What is worse is when there will be people all around us, but something has happened to make one feel fenced off. What does the doctor feel who has missed a case of meningitis; or the counsellor known to have broken confidentiality; or the priest who promised to visit, yet didn't get round to it before the parishioner died?

Such failure can be a frighteningly lonely place in which to examine oneself. There is that terrible shock when the realization of what has happened hits home. There is the anger with myself that is always part of guilt; and the resentment against the 'system' or others who may have let me down, or not saved me, or – worse – betrayed me. There is apprehension about the consequences. Maybe I realize I tried to cope too much on my own. No wonder I now feel so utterly on my own, despite expressions of support or sympathy from colleagues or loved ones.

Simon, you went to sleep on me? Can't you stick it out with me a single hour? Stay alert, be in prayer, so you don't enter the danger zone without even knowing it. Don't be naïve. Part of you is eager, ready for anything in God; another part is as lazy as an old dog sleeping by the fire.
Jesus (Mark 15.37, 38, *The Message*)

Yet the agony of loneliness can also occur to people who are in the right, saying what is true and doing what is really good. This happened in Gethsemane. How close was Jesus to resentment when, with a heavy heart, he upbraided the faithful inner core of his disciples? Can we understand how abandoned and let down he felt?

Maybe you have had an experience that identifies with that. How much of a comfort can it be to know that our Lord understands, and is in solidarity with you, as a result of his dreadful agony, which felt as though it was crushing out his life.

Maybe you know a colleague, or friend, who is feeling deeply isolated; it could be the unpopularity of the whistle-blower, or of the one who has let the side down. She or he will be feeling the condemnation of personal exclusion. Is there a way for you to communicate with her or him that includes some understanding, some solidarity?

ISOLATED

We come into the world alone; we will leave it alone. Sure, people may be around, but none can come with me.

But, Lord, that fundamental aloneness is something I am struggling with in my caring.

You come into the world alone and you go out of the world alone.
Yet it seems to me that you are more alone while living than even going and coming
Emily Carr
(1871–1945)

How wonderful it would be if those of us who care for sick family could care with other people; could we form a 'caring colony', like a big home; but we share the caring? But for now, I am alone, Lord, for most of the time. Alone with the one I care for, and with whom almost everything that can be said has been said. Help me, Lord!

And, Lord, what of the loneliness of those of us who are professionals, who have been isolated by circumstance, or who carry a heavy burden of guilt, whether warranted or not? – do you see our burden?

In every one there is a loneliness, an inner chamber of peculiar life into which God only can enter.
George Macdonald
(1824–1905)

I ache, Lord. I ache inside. Will you come into my aloneness?

I understand it, and I have known it. Even now, I feel it, as those who I call and call again turn away, and my dying and rising is as nothing to them. I know, my child.

What can I do? It seems there is nothing to
be done save to accept it, to persevere; to
grit one's teeth and go on . . .

*Yes, there is. Loneliness is a bog, a slough, and
only the light survive it. Many there are who
take it upon themselves as a cross, and those
they do meet find it laid across their shoulders
until they, too, run. And so the process con-
tinues, and the afflicted sink ever deeper into
the slough.*

Lord, I don't want that. Help me see how
to avoid it . . .

*Don't dwell on it. Love and laugh. Walk with
me, the man afflicted with sorrows, the one
esteemed stricken; yet it was your sins I carried
– alone. You will find me lightness and joy. Be
likewise. Take my yoke upon you and learn of
me, for I am meek and lowly in heart, and you
will find rest for your souls.*

You talk in Scriptures.

*Yes. They reflect my glory, and the glory of my
Father in heaven. Soak them up like a sponge;
they will lift your spirit! Look at my creation.
It will remind you of me. Don't examine your
loneliness. You will sink into it like the bog;
you will be lost. Lie on the top of it and sun
yourself!*

Will there be no burden left, O Lord?

Oh, yes. There will. But it is in acceptance-with-joy that you will overcome. And, from time to time, I will send a companion to be with you for a little while. Make them so welcome they will be looking for the opportunity to come back! But do not share your burden with any but me; only I can help you carry it.

Lord, with you I will carry this great burden. I know you understand, and I know you have the strength to help me. I look to you; grant me that patience I need, help me to turn aside the voices that tell me my life is seeping away; fill me with more and more of your life! Goodness – I think of those in solitary confinement only because they believe in you, and will not deny you! Bless them, O Lord! Be with them! Let them not despair! And of those outcast because of illness, because of appearance or disability or race; be with them! Show them your face. Oh, and the one I care for! Condemned to be with me every hour! Help that one, I pray!

Lord, I reflect; you have worked a miracle. Here I am, praying for others, and not myself! Thank you.

VALLEY OF THE SHADOW

Come to me and I will give you rest, all you who work so hard beneath a heavy yoke.

Matthew 11.28 (Living Bible)

Come aside and rest awhile.

You have seen the valley of the shadow of death; you have felt its oppression wrap itself around your heart and squeeze. The spectre of the sick has sickened you too.

And you're at the end of your tether.

So were the disciples of Jesus. Even Jesus himself.

They were utterly besieged by so many demands that they had no time even to eat.

The problem was not just the demands; it was for them too the psychological effect of suddenly seeing those normally hidden, kept in their sick room because it's too difficult to get them out – and now, look! Stretchers everywhere – so many, and so needy.

The full extent of human morbidity was revealed, and Jesus saw the disciples were overwhelmed.

Come away! – and rest awhile!
Come away! – there is no sin in it!
Come away! – the rest will reorientate you to the task you face.

There are times to take the yoke of Jesus, the yoke of gentleness and lowliness of heart, and finding his rest amid the storms.

But there are also times when nothing less than a laying down will do. Jesus will whisper the word into our hearts when that time comes.

We must not be afraid of it. Our strength is not without limit. If regular respite care, to give time aside with the Lord and those we love, is a possibility, we should enquire whether it is not a gift from the Lord's hand.

Respite restores relationship – with God, with others; and those we care for benefit even though there may be for them a cost – the cost of losing you for a little while. Yet the gain is greater.

Look for God's gift of respite times, for they complement and enable gentleness and lowliness of heart.

VALLEY OF THE SHADOW

Though I walk through the valley of the shadow of death,
I will fear no evil; for you are with me Lord,
Your rod and your staff, they comfort me.

Psalm 23 (*Common Worship*)

Are you there? I cry out, 'Is anybody there?' I feel so much on my own in this steep and terrible defile. It is a wild and fearful place, the crags hang over me – I suppose I am be-tween the rocks and a hard place. Who made me think that stupid thought? Perhaps I am not alone. Surely someone nudged me; is it you, Lord? Yes; thank God!

Lord, what a relief: I confess my fear is very insidious – per-haps I should know better; but it happens to me, creeps up on me, seems to settle round my shoulders, squeezing the confidence out of me. I do get really scared, break out in a cold sweat, as those storm clouds pile up.

Lord, in this dark and dreadful place I need to assert it: you are my Comforter and my Shepherd! There, I have said it; thank you for the will that informs my words. Certainly my heart needs to be trusting and hopeful, Lord, sure of your presence and your protection. I want to let the truth sink into my soul: '. . . *you are with me, Lord.*'

As a good shepherd, you would go all the way to protect me, risking your life to fight off snarling lions and howling wolves. I do believe you went all the way: you did, you gave up your life to set me free. Lord, this gives me a feeling of space. Before, I was constrained, as though I had no freedom of movement. Now I can relax, breathe deep – it is like your Spirit is breathed into me. I am glad, I praise you, for all you have done to sustain and refresh me. It is really true: Lord, where you guide, you provide.

I realize, thanks to you, my Lord, that although I am still overshadowed it is safe to climb onward. I bid you, fulfil your promises:

- Sustain and nourish me, especially whenever the old enemy is prowling round, like a roaring lion, seeking for someone to devour.
- Like a good shepherd, smoothing in the healing oil, soothing the lamb who has had a really scratchy time in a tangled thicket. Let me feel your healing touch, your anointing to re-consecrate me to your purposes.
- Let your blessings overflow, like a chalice that never empties.
- Let the angels of goodness, kindness and loving mercy be with me wherever I go. Then shall I know, that you are with me, letting me dwell with you: '. . . *in your house for ever.*'

So, Lord, I rejoice before you: I know beyond all doubt – in body and soul, heart and mind – you have been faithful, granting that prayer I have made thousands of times:

Lighten our darkness, we beseech thee, O Lord; and by thy great mercy defend us from all the perils and dangers of this night; for the love of thy only Son, our Saviour, Jesus Christ. Amen.

Book of Common Prayer

THE SHEPHERD

Paul Gallico, in his rather mystical book, *The Shepherd*, tells a story of a jet fighter pilot lost in mist, with his radio systems broken down, late on Christmas Eve. Out of nowhere an ancient Mosquito appears at his wing tip and guides him right down to the runway, where the landing lights come on despite the base being closed for Christmas. There is of course more to the story.

I am the good shepherd; I know my own and my own know me, as the Father knows me and I know the Father; and I lay down my life for the sheep.
Jesus (John 10.14)

There have been times when I have felt lost, and seemed unable to get help. I needed a shepherd good enough to find me and guide me to safety.

In World War 2 any ship straggling behind a convoy could be in grave danger from a U-boat wolf pack. The corvette or frigate sent to pick up such a ship was known as a shepherd.

For thus says the Lord God: I myself will search for my sheep, and will seek them out.
Ezekiel 34.11

There have been times when I have fallen behind and have been in danger of sinking, overwhelmed by all that is happening. I needed a shepherd good enough to find me, stay with me and protect me.

On a farm in North Devon it was a privilege to spend a day with a shepherd. Clearly he knew his sheep individually, though they all looked much the same to me. Letting the sheepdogs out of the Land-Rover he drove slowly forward while 150 sheep were herded into a corner. He needed to give an injection to one of them. Taking the syringe he plunged into the herd and moved directly to that particular sheep, to bring the means of healing.

There have been times when I have been in need of help and healing though in the middle of a crowd of good folk, who seemed unable to help. I needed a shepherd good enough to recognize me and able to meet my need.

As shepherds seek out their flocks when they are among their scattered sheep, so I will seek out my sheep.
I will rescue them from all the places to which they have been scattered . . .
Ezekiel 34.12

We value the icon of the loving shepherd. Though we often think of ourselves as called to the role of the shepherd, we have to learn that we too need the Good Shepherd to find, meet, protect, feed, sustain and guide us into the safety of his keeping. Then we realize again that he did always care and was totally capable of doing all those things and much more for us – even gave his life to complete the job.

I myself will be the shepherd of my sheep . . . says the Lord God
. . . I will bind up the injured, and I will strengthen the weak . . .
Ezekiel 34.15, 16

Perhaps I can stop bleating about the bush, recover confidence, and be ready to renew my other vocation: like being one of the sheepdogs, guiding and helping sheep into fulfilling the purposes of the Good Shepherd.

And you are my sheep, the sheep of my pasture, and I am your God, says the Lord God.
Ezekiel 34.31

THE SHEPHERD

I am a carer. I'm not allowed to be sick.

I look after the sick! Me: I have to be eternally strong; a rock.

The trouble is, Lord, that I too need healing. Be my shepherd, ready to identify me as the one needing attention, ready to come to me to administer what is necessary. (An aside, I'm not too keen on needles. I prefer the laying-on-of-hands, if that's alright.)

Sometimes, Lord, my pains aren't visible. How will you notice? You will anyway? Well, that's comforting.

Suppose it's a deep-inside pain – not even physical? You'll see that, too? I understand (well – I'm trying to). And will you help me with that?

What if it's spiritual? What if it's something in my relationship with you? What then? What if it's something I'm caught in – a sin of some sort; what then? You're good with sins? But I must bring it into the light. Your light.

Now say no more: listen to me for a while – you talk and talk and talk! Anyone would think you didn't understand that prayer is a two-way thing. Now listen . . .

The shepherd loves his sheep, if he's a good

shepherd. I am The Good Shepherd. My sheep hear my voice, and I keep each one safe. You are my sheep – you, singular – and you belong to my flock. And I love you.

I train you to be dependent on me. The world trains you to be independent; but never was a sheep independent, and it is not my purpose that you should be so. You are made for fellowship with me, and it is as you come to see your need of me moment by moment, day by day, that the fellowship grows. Sometimes I shall be behind you; sometimes alongside you. And on occasions I shall be before you, and you will see me, and rejoice.

Always I am there, never more than a call away. Usually, my sheep behave as though it were not so, and complain that I am 'distant'. I am not distant. Rather you are distant; you dwell in your thoughts in a foreign land where I am not. I am, I AM, in my Kingdom. If you acknowledge me as King then you are my subject. And I am close.

I have a great need for Christ; I have a great Christ for my need.
Charles Haddon Spurgeon
(1834–92)

But remember; I am a loving King who washes feet and binds up hearts.

Amen. Oh, amen! Wash my feet and bind my heart, O King Jesus. I bow before your throne.

Be thou before me and behind, on the left and the right, above and below.
Heal me, O Lord, and I shall be healed indeed (from Jeremiah 17.14). Amen.

ENCOURAGEMENT

This is my commandment, that you love one another as I have loved you

John 15.12

By this will all know that you are my disciples; if you have love for one another.

John 13.35

What encouragement is there for us in our caring?

Caring is hard work; it's laying down your life; it's having to keep going when your body tells you it's had enough. Where's the encouragement?

I don't know. One thing I do know, though. When even we as mere mortals see a life laid down for others, when we see a life lost in serving, our hearts leap. We know something of the *divine* response to the selflessness of giving and serving within ourselves; we seem to react like God does.

We may fear being called to care selflessly ourselves, but, when we see others doing it, we honour their example.

We need to see that example as encouragement. When we look at the sacrifices of others, we see the value and beauty of

You came here to serve, not to rule.
Thomas à Kempis
(*c.*1380–1471)

self-giving very clearly. When we are called to make such a sacrifice ourselves, we are more inclined to focus on bewailing the loss of our freedom; to wonder if the sacrifice is a waste of our life.

Look at the extreme; Mother Teresa. Was hers a wasted life? Few would think so.

She carried a serenity in her caring, the serenity of knowing she was called to care for those who no one else cared about – except God. So she worked in his name.

And she exuded something special as a result. A serenity, a warmth of manner and a sense of humour – reflected in a sparkle of manner, a twinkle of eye.

So it is with other carers who seem to have grasped at a meaning, a deeper meaning, in their care.

God is where my helplessness begins.
Oswald Chambers
(1874–1917)

They are not overcome by their caring. There is enough of them not to be sucked dry. Perhaps more accurately, they have found inner resources that meet their need. Indeed, they often seem to be well resourced both internally and externally.

May you in your caring also find this inner resourcing from the Lord himself, together with the outer resourcing of help, training and respite, and of encouragement and friendship.

ENCOURAGEMENT

*I pray that . . . he may grant that you may be
strengthened
in your inner being with power through his
Spirit,
and that Christ may dwell in your hearts
through faith,
as you are being rooted and grounded in love.*

Ephesians 3.16, 17

Holy God, holy and true, holy and strong,
I thank you for your call to acts of care and
concern, reflecting your holy compassion.

This service that I offer in your name, O
holy One, is not, I trust, an idea I dreamed
up but the carrying out of your holy will.

*I can do all things
through him who
strengthens me.
In any case it was
kind of you to
share my distress.*
Philippians 4.13,
14

Is that why, holy Lord, this caring is so
worthwhile, and the inspiration from
others is so buoyant, uplifting and
strengthening?

Holy God, I praise you for the example
of many brave souls, who blazed a trail
of new and inspiring works, and who
encourage me to give my all.

To share the hope of that greater company
who have steadfastly trod your way, holy
Lord, builds up a mutual trust in your
guidance.
It is your courage, Holy Jesus, that I
perceive in them.

*I give you thanks,
O Lord, with my
whole heart;
before the gods I
sing your praise.
On the day
I called you
answered me,
you increased my
strength of soul.*
Psalm 138.1, 3

I thank you that you can use it to encourage me, building up my heart to be brave and true.

Holy Father, pray answer my call to you now: in your great and holy compassion, reach out to those who need encouraging. Aware of many, in my heart I lift them to you:

The faint-hearted, and the weak willed, those easily frightened or prey to addictions; some overwhelmed by the dreariness of the same old lonely duties of care day by day, with no respite in sight; others having no one with whom to share, or enduring relentless pains and anguish;
and all for whom the seemingly endless battles with bureaucracy or budgeting drain away their eagerness.

Holy Spirit, holy and good, holy and merciful, let the words of St Peter come true:

*And after you have suffered for a little while,
the God of all grace, who has called you to his
eternal glory in Christ,
will himself restore, support, strengthen and
establish you.
To him be the power for ever and ever. Amen.*

1 Peter 5.10, 11

ASSURANCE

*All shall be well; and all manner of things
shall be well.*

Lady Julian of Norwich

There are moments when we feel a gentle glow of satisfaction and relief as something turns out well: we see recovery begin, distress melting away, smiles appearing, a load lightening; and the sun shines brightly. It is a rewarding experience, whether we feel we have deserved it or not. We can be glad and share in the growth of joy and gratitude in the people for whom we care.

These are moments when sharing in the fruits of healing, in those whom we serve, brings healing to our souls. Confidence grows – doubts are allayed. Anxieties are replaced by calm. Space suddenly appears in the midst of hassle. Conviction grows – we are moving in the right direction, and our vocation is being fulfilled.

We know that all things work together for good for those who love God, who are called according to his purpose.
Romans 8.28

There are moments when we feel particularly welcome in a team. Recognition and inclusion seem to be assured. Our skills and contributions are openly valued. To know that we are fully accepted and belong adds meaning to our work and enhances all that we offer. Caring then feels much more worthwhile; we can be rightly glad about that.

God tested them and found them worthy of himself.
Wisdom of Solomon 3.4

There are moments when failures in the past are absolved. It may be a formal matter of confessing sins, owning up to mistakes, pleading guilty to errors and omissions. It is certainly a great relief when all is worked through; we feel released, even forgiven and accepted despite what happened. Reconciliation and redemption are at the heart of the gospel. When our neighbour answers the call to be reconciled to us we are all in a better, more comfortable place.

There are moments when the appreciation we receive is warm and deep. Gratitude expressed, care acknowledged, help valued, all adds up to thankfulness on both sides. Of course we can take joy and delight in this. It is more than just being 'all in a day's work'; even if it did seem a humdrum, oft-repeated intervention at the time. Appreciation is an action of grace in what can so easily be a one-sided relationship.

God arranged that some received the reward of their labours even before they had set to work, others while they were still working, and others again at the time of their death.
Reader, ask yourself, which of them was made more humble.
John Climacus (died 649)

These are all moments to treasure, for they are part of the redemption of times of frustration, failure or helplessness. Such moments can run into one another, even if there are very hard things also going on. They become part of the totality of knowing an unconditional love at work in us – a love greater than we possess or can imagine, yet which allows us to rejoice in the experience of true wholeness.

ASSURANCE

My Father

Thank you for those times when I know that all is well.

Thank you for the times when all my caring, all my labouring, bears fruit and I can, as it were, eat of that fruit and enjoy it.

Thank you for the times when my contribution is recognized, when I am valued.

Thank you for the times when I am at peace with my neighbour, my family, the world.

God takes life's pieces and gives us unbroken peace.
W. D. Gough

Thank you for the wonder of forgiving and being forgiven.

It is well, it is well with my soul.

Yet I know that it will not always be so: I am fickle, others are fickle – only you are not. Even you seem to be from time to time, though I know that reveals only that I am 'looking through a glass darkly'.

*Joy is sorrow
inside out;
Grief remade
again.*
Hannah Hurnard
(1905–90)

Help me not only to bask in this assurance that all is well, but to remember it . . .

. . . so that next time I doubt you, I shall have an even stronger case for dismissing the thought.

Help me to live in your presence, where light is; and help me to do all things as though I were doing them for you, with a willing heart and with joy.

But for tonight, grant me the sleep of the fulfilled, for that is how I feel.

It is well, it is well with my soul. Amen.

PRAYING

Prayer is weakness leaning on omnipotence.

W. S. Bowden

Seven days without prayer makes one weak.

Allen E. Bartlett

God knows how weak we are.
Jesus shared that very weakness, that very limitation, albeit without sin.
But he knows our situation; and that knowing should be for us a great encouragement.

If we are weak, as we are, we need all the help we can get;
And, since God hears our prayers, and is always within reach of us,
And since he is omnipotent (unlike me),
There is a certain logic to reflecting our weaknesses and our struggles to him,
And asking for his help in them.

You need not cry very loud; he is nearer to us than we think.
Brother Lawrence
(1605–91)

When we also remember that he loves us, there is even more basis for such recourse to him.

The problem with prayer is that when we most need to be doing it we least feel like doing it.

*Don't pray
when you feel
like it. Have an
appointment with
the Lord and
keep it. A man is
powerful on his
knees.*
Corrie Ten Boom
(1892–1983)

That is why prayer may need to be disciplined until such time as it is automatic, and we truly 'pray at all times', as the apostle Paul exhorts.

But the important thing is never to wait to pray. There is no better time than now, and no better place than where you are.

There is a joy in prayer, especially the prayer that arises from our lips reluctantly, because we have felt unworthy in some way.

*Never wait for
fitter time or place
to talk to the Lord.
To wait till you go
to church, or to
your room, is to
make him wait.
He will listen as
you walk.*
George Macdonald
(1824–1905)

It is an indication to the Lord that our heart's desire is to keep in communion with him, and that is something he always seems to bless.

So we must remember to pray often, especially when things have gone wrong and, as a consequence, so have we. Prayer changes things – yes. But it also changes us; and then we change things.

PRAYING

Our Father, who art in heaven, hallowed be thy name;

Heavenly Father, reverently, with adoration I come.
Though I praise you alone, I never pray on my own, but
always as one of the company of your faithful people on
earth, the body of Christ; and with all those witnesses
around your throne, where he for ever offers intercession
for us.

Thy kingdom come; thy will be done; on earth as it is in heaven.

Holy Father, aware of your sovereign rule, living the
kingdom, we dedicate our prayer, obedient to your will
– confessing how often we put our desires first.
In your mercy, open our minds and hearts to your will;
open our eyes to see this world as you see it; looking upon
your children as you do, understanding their deepest needs
in the way you love.
By the inspiration of your Holy Spirit grant us the
perspective that sees earth in relation to heaven.

Give us this day our daily bread.

Fatherly God, looking at those for whom we pray,
informed by your vision, purposes and wisdom, and
standing in-between, we bring them before you.
As you created us, Father, and clothed Jesus in flesh, so we
pray, trusting you meet bodily needs: –
feed the hungry – comfort the sorrowing –
restore health and joy – give freedom for the addicted –

justice for the oppressed – and peace of mind for the
disturbed.
Yet even as we lift them, and so many to you, as we must,
we realize you already have taken steps to provide:
we thank you for the signs of your healing salvation.

And forgive us our trespasses, as we forgive those who trespass
against us.

Eternal Father, mighty to save, by the sacrifice of Jesus –
through whose wounds you released your healing mercy –
bring us the grace of forgiveness and reconciliation.
Help each of us to grasp hold of this opportunity, to say:
'I forgive: despite the pain I've suffered I will love you –
or at least treat you as if I love you.'
At all those times when truth dictates I need to say sorry,
let me humbly accept the word of forgiveness.
In this, we praise you for your patience, mercy and love.

And lead us not into temptation; but deliver us from evil.

Almighty Father, we and those we love, or for whom we
care, need your protection and defence against the wiles
of evil; pray let your holy angels guard us from all the
dangers: temptations, at the low ebb, in slippery places,
undermined.
Father, call to us, strengthen us, guide us, hold us, lead us
and bring us safely to that haven, that heaven you intend
for us.

For thine is the kingdom, the power and the glory, for ever and
ever. Amen.

RECONCILIATION

> *Strange to see how a good dinner and feasting*
> *reconciles everybody.*
>
> Samuel Pepys

A good meal together offers recognition and inclusion. It helps us relax, feel at peace within and thus outwardly peaceful to others. Good examples of this can be seen in some movies; who could forget the melting of the icy emotional reserve of the Danish villagers in *Babette's Feast*? A more recent and equally moving example is *Chocolat*, again about the struggle for the acceptance of the stranger. Nearer home, all those who have been on an Alpha course know just how important the meal is in building the group and the fellowship, making folk receptive to one another.

Celebrating a feast, Jesus chose to make a meal into a greater celebration – to be a foretaste of the heavenly banquet, that moment when reconciliation with God and others will be complete. To celebrate the Eucharist, to share in the Lord's Supper, to receive Holy Communion, are moments of the deepest consciousness of being at one and at peace with God. People need the reconciliation found at the heart of the Gospel.

In the world of giving and receiving care the moments of human reconciliation may be more obvious where the relationship is with family or friends. It just doesn't seem to happen that professionals feast with their patients or clients – though pastors may do with parishioners. But do we need 'Reconciliation' in these caring contexts? Sadly, sometimes we do; maybe with clients, maybe with working colleagues.

What is more common is that receivers look for human kindness and empathy from their professional carers. When it is offered it is gladly recognized. In an age when Health and Social services are under pressure we can all suffer the effects, either in the care we receive or in our working situation. How can we share what the other suffers? How can we prevent any breakdown in communications brought about by being trapped in dire straits? Perhaps we have to be imaginative in reaching out to express our solidarity.

Some twenty years ago there was a time of great tension in central Europe. Before *perestroika* the Iron Curtain was real. At one of the road crossings a British army patrol found itself opposite a Russian patrol. Both sides were armed to the teeth. Only a white line painted across the road separated them. There was silence. Who would turn away first? The English corporal asked his men a question; one produced a new pack of Marlboro cigarettes. The corporal put it on the ground by the white line, and with his boot pushed it over the line for the Russian corporal to pick it up. Each Russian took one cigarette, and the pack was returned, in the same way, still containing enough cigarettes for the British.

This was a feast-like gesture of reconciling solidarity, expressed by both sides, in a world full of danger. We are all in this together: we need to be at peace with one another. 'Blessed are the peacemakers,' said Jesus.

RECONCILIATION

Lord, I want to work through what we considered this morning.

If I were the soldier facing the white line, what would I want to do?

Yes, I would push the cigarettes over. But how I would love to do more!

How I would love to have (imagining myself being there) approached the white line with my weapon left on the ground, and my hands open and empty.

And have extended my hand across the line of hostility. How I would have prayed that a Russian soldier would have taken it, and embraced me; because I am human too, and we have no quarrel. Not he and I.

I would have wept. But is that a sign of weakness, Lord? I think not.

I remember the story of the Christmas football game between men intent the day before on killing one another, during World War 1. Let me be a peacemaker!

I remember the courage of David Attenborough as a young man, striding with a smile towards a group of hostile-looking natives with his hand outstretched, as though he were meeting a business associate at Victoria Station. Let me, too, be a peacemaker!

Help me to see things from the other point of view. Forgive me for demonizing men and women for no good reason. I want to be a peacemaker.

I don't want to say 'Peace, peace!' when there is no peace. But I do want to reach across the divides of prejudice and love-lessness with something of the warmth of your love incarnate in me.

Thank you for the many who both agree and act accordingly. Thank you for the love that flows. Just help me to play my part too, I pray; to see behind the veil to the problems that those who don't provide good service are up against. Let me be sympathetic and understanding.

And so let more of your love flow in reconciliation in every area that I, as a carer, come across, and let your name be glorified. Amen.

SIGNS OF HEALING

*From the bitterness of disease, man learns the
sweetness of health.*

Spanish proverb

*It would be a
blessing if each
human being were
stricken blind and
deaf for a few
days at some time
during his adult
life. Darkness
would make him
more appreciative
of sight; silence
would teach him
the joys of sound.*
Helen Keller
(1880–1968)

Healing is sometimes a subtle thing.

It can be the difference between a sigh and a sniff when food is brought.

It can be the difference between disinterest and interest in family news.

It can be the difference between a joke ignored and a joke appreciated.

It can be entirely physical, but more commonly it's a whole-of-person thing.

We all know it, for we all recognize when we 'get our energy back' after a viral illness.

Healing is sometimes expected – like when we get a bug; we anticipate a full recovery.

In people with chronic illness, it is not always the case: there are many much more complex factors that can precipitate a decline – anything from something particularly depressing on the news ('I think I've lived long enough'), to a tragedy or a shame, in the family ('I never thought I'd live to see *that*'), to the clinical state of depression, to a simple infection, such as a waterworks infection. The key is to make the diagnosis accurately, treat appropriately at whatever level of the being we need to, and pray.

First signs of healing, when they come, are often exciting. Possibilities for the future occur to us, possibilities for the one we are caring for and for ourselves – possibilities that perhaps we had assumed would never again present themselves. God has an ongoing plan. But we shall not presume upon the future again, and we may find ourselves asking what the meaning for the healing is. Healing for what?

The day after Dorothy Kerin, founder of Burrswood, was miraculously healed of tubercular meningitis in 1912, her doctor was summoned. He assumed it was to sign her death certificate, so ill had she been. When he saw her restored, running up and down stairs and with all her emaciation gone, he held his head in his hands and said, 'Great God, what is the meaning of this?' The question is a good one for us to ask when we see healing taking place, even if it is a little less dramatic. What is God saying, what is he wanting? I do not have the answer, but it will help us to reflect that question to God.

SIGNS OF HEALING

Verses from Psalm 103

Bless the Lord, O my soul,
and all that is within me bless his holy name.

Lord, with a joyful heart I bless you;
and not just with my heart, wonderful
    saviour,
but with every fibre of my being –
singing your praise in body and soul,
rejoicing in the depths of my spirit.

Bless the Lord, O my soul,
and forget not all his benefits;

Over and over again, dear Lord,
I am reminded of your promises being
    kept,
of your purposes unfolding day by day
just as, through your holy prophets,
you said it would be when your Spirit,
O Lord God, anoints your chosen ones.

Who forgives all your sins
and heals all your infirmities.

Yes, Lord, we bless you and thank you
for all the signs of your working in us.
Your moving among us is good news
for those who are oppressed, or hurting,
as we see broken hearts soothed, restored;
and witness your people freed from the
    disease that has held them captive.

Who redeems your life from the pit
and crowns you with faithful love and
compassion.

Our praises rise to you, Lord of all
   compassion,
You restore again the chance of fulfilling
   your will –
in our lives and in our loving, knowing
   your ways –
seeing again all your desires for us
and our loved ones, all for whom you
   care,
all with whom we share your works and
   goodness.

Who satisfies you with good things,
so that your youth is restored like an eagle's.

It matters not, O Lord, whether the healing
is of symptoms relieved, cure received,
or the sustaining strength that gives faith,
hope and grace to live and bless you
despite enduring disability or frailty.
In every case we bless you for your mercy,
for the comfort that lovingly carries us
and keeps us joyful in your healing
   presence.
Bless you, Lord, bless you, bless you.

Bless the Lord, all you his hosts.
You ministers of his that do his will.

GROWTH ENABLED

*And other seed fell into good soil and brought
forth grain, growing up
and increasing and yielding thirty and sixty
and a hundredfold.*

Jesus (Mark 4.8)

Growth is natural and we expect it. The
seed we sow is made to germinate; the
plant we see growing is doing the only
thing it can. We are keen to tend it and find
joy in witnessing the growth. If the growth
needs our provisioning and enabling, as
in that of a baby, and then the child, we
rightly take great delight in the growth,
and in the hints of maturity to come. We
are concerned not merely with physical
growth, but with realizing the exciting
potential of mental, emotional, relational
and spiritual development.

*God made man
lord of the earth,
but he was small
and but a child.
He had to grow
and reach full
maturity.*
Bishop Irenaeus
(130–202)

In the parable of the sower Jesus took
great care to highlight the various physical
hindrances there might be to the process
from seed to fruitfulness. The explanation
of the parable we are given in the Gospel
interprets those hindrances in terms that
include threats, the will, the emotions,
distractions and other tribulations. In our
work of caring many of us seem frequently
to be dealing with what hinders people
from achieving full maturity.

*Every painful
event contains
within itself a seed
of growth and
liberation.*
Anthony de Mello
(Indian Jesuit)

The vocation to deal with hindrances, adversity and pain is very special indeed just when it comes to being involved with enabling growth. What a privilege it is to be with a patient, client, parishioner or loved one just at the moment where the overcoming of a disability or an affliction heralds the flowering of life's possibilities. Whether it is a first-time discovery, or growth restored after hope seemed slim, it is a joy to be able to share in what has happened. Our work and care then feels very rewarding.

*Happy events
make life
delightful but
they do not lead
to self-discovery
and growth and
freedom.
That privilege is
reserved to the
things and persons
and situations that
cause us pain.*
Anthony de Mello

We, the carers, also need to be growing. Our growth and self-discovery also comes through the people and situations that cause us pain. We are unlikely to welcome that at the time. We, too, have to accept that we need someone, or some others, who can help and lead us through the pain to the gain. Whether we call these enabling angels our family, support group, supervisor, soul friend or spiritual director matters little. What matters is being ready to take the humble step of accepting such nurture. Then we become open to producing a rich harvest in our souls. In thankfulness, we shall want to continue sustaining that maturity.

*Riches are gotten
with pain,
kept with care and
lost with grief.*
Richard Fuller
(1608–61)

My Lord and my God: I do not like pain.
I never coped well with the pain of others, and I do not relish it myself.
Funny it is that some seem almost to find an identity in it.
Not me. Perhaps, if it's OK by you, Lord, I prefer to find my identity in my hobby, my family, my sense of humour; but not pain. No thanks.

I did hope you might want to find your identity in me.

Lord! I do! Forgive me! I thought the very fact that I was praying showed that!

Praying? Oh, I thought you were complaining. I accept your apology and I forgive you. I always do.
If I shared my wisdom with you, would you listen?

Would I listen! Of course I would listen!

Ponder on Jesus for a while. What were the hallmarks of his life?

Love. I think he laughed a lot, too. And, I guess one has to add, suffered.

One does have to add it, yes. His willingness to undergo suffering for you was what made me so thrilled with him. I didn't make him do that . . .

It's wonderful. Um . . . where's this leading?

Though he was a son, yet he learned obedience by the things

*which he suffered; and, having been perfected, he became the
author of eternal salvation to all who obey him . . .*

You're quoting the letter to the Hebrews.

*Yes. It is my word. Listen and learn. I make you grow through
suffering. When my people suffered, they came to me. When they
grew sleek and fat, they rebelled. They thought their sleekness
was all their own work. But they all became food for worms in
the end.*

I'm not sure I am following.

*True. When you identify with my Son, I bless you. Everything of
his, I bless. When you love as he loves, when you laugh for joy of
him, when you suffer for his sake and the sake of the gospel, my
love pours upon you in great rivers; I boast of you before heaven
– he is mine, I say – see how he follows! Remember how proud I
was of Job? Can you believe I boast of you?*

But I complain!

*So the devil reminds me. But that's only some of the time. I call
you to my side, I restrain you lovingly from what takes you away,
I gently test you. And now I am encouraging you. Don't give up!
You do well, and I love you. I also test you. Be encouraged. Encourage the one you care for too.*

This is a wonder. My Lord, take me and use me as you
choose. Just stay close at least when I need you.

*I will. Look unto me and be radiant! That is my word to you. Look
unto me and be radiant.*

Amen. I will! Thank you, Lord. Grant us sleep now, I pray,
and strength for the morrow . . .
Amen.

THE THANK YOUS

For all that has been, thanks!
For all that shall be, yes!

Dag Hammarskjöld, 1905–61

So the healing has happened. Who was responsible?

Sometimes that is hard to say. Usually it's a combination of care and prayer, medicine and ministry; for though medicine alone may produce a cure, it less frequently produces a healing.

A healing leads to something. A cure does not always do so. A healing usually affects the whole person. A cure does not always do so. When the whole person is affected, we may well see new perspectives, new love, and new understanding following. Indeed, in some ways a healing without change is a shame. Healing should promote enquiry – for what have I been healed? And that question may embrace the carer as well.

Thanks are appropriate, and may be forthcoming. Wise professional carers hold such thanks lightly, for they recognize that their

*Some hae meat
and canna eat,
And some would
eat that want it;
But we hae meat
and we can eat –
And so the Lord be
thank-ed!*
Robert Burns
(1759–96)

care may have played only a limited role in the process of healing; notwithstanding, thanks are always a huge encouragement to a caring team.

A loving family who have expended much in practical care will also find great blessing in carefully and thoughtfully expressed thanks, or even a straightforward 'thank you for what you've done for me'; but they may have to accept something less with sweetness. There is an eternal reward. Not every person who has found healing has the insight to see the sacrifices that have been made on their behalf.

It is right, too, that God be thanked in some meaningful way. We remember the story of the lepers to whom Jesus ministered; one is commended for returning to give thanks. It was the Samaritan. He gave thanks, and worshipped.

*And Peter's
mother-in-law
was sick with a
great fever, and
they besought him
for her. And he
stood over her and
rebuked the fever;
and it left her:
and immediately
she rose up and
ministered unto
them.*
Luke 4.38b, 39

Those who receive much, love much, Jesus tells us; and loving Jesus much leads to an inclination to follow him. Hence a life can change – even a committed life, committed to Christ, can find new depths of devotion and obedience, having known God's healing and forgiveness. 'I must have got better for a purpose', people will say. And so the carer and the one cared for may both be able to ask, 'Lord, what can I now do for you?' It is a part of our thanks to him.

THE THANK YOUS

This is the day that you have made, O Lord;
we will rejoice and be glad in it.
You are my God and I will thank you;
you are my God and I will exalt you.

Psalm 118.24, 28

Early in the morning, O Father of all mercies,
I take account of your goodness and generosity.
Deliberately I become aware of your good will,
of all good gifts, the nice things, the blessings,
even the challenges that call forth your grace.
There is so much for which to be thankful.

We . . . give you most humble and hearty thanks
for all your goodness and loving kindness.
We bless you for our creation, preservation,
and all the blessings of this life . . .

Today, Father, in these my thanksgivings
I want to concentrate on the gift of gratitude.
Over and over again I find myself valuing
all the thank yous that come my way.
The appreciation makes such a difference –
enhances relationships in clinic, parish or family.

. . . but above all for your immeasurable love
in the redemption of the world by our Lord Jesus Christ,
for the means of grace, and for the hope of glory.

Yes, generous Father, we bless you and thank you
for all the signs of appreciation in our family circle.

Sometimes it may be just a word, a smile, a sign
whose meaning we have grown to recognize.
Such expressions give a sense of thankfulness
and well-being about the love that is between us.

And give us, we pray, such a sense of all your mercies
that our hearts may be unfeignedly thankful . . .

How can we best express our thankfulness?
Father, I wish to convey, assert, confirm
all in me that responds gladly and warmly to your grace.
Surely it is to be more than merely saying, 'Thank you'.

. . . and that we show forth your praise
not only with our lips but in our lives . . .

May it be a sacrifice of thanksgiving,
in actions that show change and growth.
Let thankfulness be part of our deeper being,
going beyond what we say to what we are.
Then, whatever happens, we can offer each day:
thankful to live within your gracious providence.

. . . by giving up ourselves to your service,
and by walking before you in holiness
and righteousness all the days of our life;
through Jesus Christ our Lord. Amen
All responses are from General Thanksgiving, ASB

GOOD OUTCOMES

*Rejoice always, pray without ceasing, give
thanks in all circumstances;
for this is the will of God in Christ Jesus for
you.*

1 Thessalonians 5.17, 18

Rewards come in various ways, and only some of them are financial. Meeting other people's needs is generally reckoned to bring deep rewards. It is very satisfying when good outcomes happen to the people we serve. When they make their gratitude clear, person to person, that is even more rewarding and encouraging. When someone deliberately comes back to say thank you that is exceptionally gratifying. So we can understand how Jesus felt when the one of the ten who had been lepers returned, praising God for his healing.

*And Jesus said
unto him, 'Arise,
go thy way; thy
faith hath made
thee whole.'*
Luke 17.19 (AV)

Such an encounter can be amazing. After a service an elderly lady came up to me in the porch of the Church of Christ the Healer at Burrswood and told me part of her story. Ten days before, her GP had found indications that her cancer had returned, and had arranged for her to go to the hospital. Before she went she had come to Burrswood, and anonymously received the laying-on-of-hands with prayer from

me, at the regular service. Now she had returned a week later to give thanks, for the
hospital had been unable to find any trace
of cancer. 'Keep praising God', I said; not
wishing to affirm or deny a miracle – far
better to keep your eyes upon Jesus.

In the language of today it feels more
comfortable to acknowledge many marvellous and wonderful things happening.
Certainly they are observed frequently in
the Burrswood hospital wing, and through
the counselling care offered. This is true in
many other places. There are times when
patients, clients, parishioners and relatives
do really well, beyond predictions. Some
seem to heal quicker; some seem to get to
the root of their emotions in remarkable
ways. Therapy and ministry are welcomed
at deep levels. Although there is much
that can be called 'cause and effect' in the
services we offer, can we not rightly rejoice
at better-than-expected outcomes?

Rejoicing like this is not the same as taking the credit. But it is right to take credit
where it is due. We should not dismiss
our part, even if we believe that it is by the
work of the Holy Spirit within us. What is
important is to be ready to recognize what
is happening, and to be glad. We wonder
– we marvel . . . Jesus spoke of 'signs' of
God's working; sometimes 'signs' are only
seen with the eye of faith.

In the Anglican report, *A Time to Heal*, (Church House Publishing, 2000) the following definition is considered:

> So a healing miracle might be defined as an inexplicable cure which, seen with the eye of faith, itself builds up faith: *inexplicable* because at that time and in those circumstances it is beyond scientific explanation; *seen with the eye of faith* because without faith it can be explained away; *builds up faith* because it should result in giving glory to God (the effect of New Testament miracles).

So when good outcomes, heartfelt thanks and even marvels appear before us should not our response be to pass on the thanks – giving glory to the author of all good gifts. Giving thanks and praise, just as the tenth leper did, confirms the prospect of wholeness.

GOOD OUTCOMES

*When good outcomes, heartfelt thanks and
even marvels appear before us, should not
our response be to pass on the thanks – giving
glory to the author of all good gifts?*

Lord, help me to see the marvels. I am
inclined to think of marvels as being the
physical things. But is it not a marvel also
when that great enemy, death, feared for
all ages, is approached in peace? Indeed it
is: hallelujah!

Is it not a marvel that death has lost its
sting, that Jesus has paid the price for my
sins, that I might be forgiven even as I turn
to him? Indeed it is: hallelujah!

*Without faith man
becomes sterile,
hopeless, and afraid
to the very core of his
being.*
Erich Fromm
(1900–80)

Is it not a marvel that the one torn by anxiety and care, paralysed by assuming burdens too great, is released into peace and
gentle submission to your purpose? Indeed it is: hallelujah!

Is it not a marvel that the one held in grief
or loss hears the call to move on, and feels
the arms of Jesus all around, sustaining
and comforting? Indeed it is: hallelujah!

Is it not a marvel that the one embittered
by the exhaustion of Chronic Fatigue
Syndrome has started to recover? – And

is walking a few steps further each week?
– And is resting with Jesus rather than
feeling left behind, bereft? Indeed it is:
hallelujah!

Lord! – help me to see the marvels! Give to
me the eye of faith, that I might see, and let
my faith be encouraged in the very seeing;
and may it be built up as I glorify you for
what I see.

*You both precede
and follow
me, and place
your hand of
blessing upon
my head. This
is too glorious,
too wonderful to
believe!*
Psalm 139.5, 6

I had not fully realized that all healing
comes from you. Even what the doctors
do. Doctors clear the obstacles to healing;
but you create us in such a way that we
then heal. What a wonder! Hallelujah!

And thank you too for what you teach us
through the sick, the infirm, the aged. In
truth, we live in a state of mutual depend-
ence, and you smile upon that as the love
of caring flows. Thank you that depend-
ence isn't a dirty word. You, Lord Jesus,
were dependent upon your Father; the
one I care for is dependent upon me, and
I am utterly dependent upon you. My next
breath is in your hands – here it comes!
– thank you, Lord.

And so in thanks and praise I run and
spread my wings and launch myself to rise
in currents of your love; I rise, I soar, and
buoyed by Spirit's lift I leave the earth-
bound far behind, to find your nearer

presence – in this life. There is no worry here – why worry? God is greater; there is no fear here – what can separate us from the love of Christ? Can sickness? Can storm? Can circumstance? Nothing can separate us from the love of God in Christ Jesus. All praise and glory be to him, for ever and ever! Amen.

REDEMPTION GLIMPSED

The strangest truth of the gospel is that redemption comes through suffering.

Milo L. Chapman

Redemption is what happens when something that we had lost control over is bought back. Hence, when finances allow, we redeem a watch from a pawn shop. It was sold; it is bought back.

It is good for us to remember, at the end of these meditations and prayers, that there is a hard truth to Christian faith.

It is this. Though we were created for fellowship with God, we quickly fell from the heights for which God had planned us, and found ourselves in slavery to sin. But the joy, of course, is that Jesus Christ came to redeem us, to pay the price to buy us back.

It was a path of suffering, a path to the Cross. But it was a path which leads us into fellowship with God not just for these three score years and ten that we may live, but for eternity. This is the redemption plan; it is the restoration of that for which God created us.

Paradoxically, it is in *our* suffering, and that of those we love, that we see more clearly God's great plan of redemption for us. Were we all in a state of unrelieved blessedness, we would slip into living for ourselves all too easily.

Never once is God said to be reconciled to man; it is always man who is reconciled to God.
William Barclay
(1907–78)

But God didn't create us to live for ourselves. We are his, and were created for fellowship with him – men and women in fellowship with God. But this is not a fellowship of equals, and God wants us to trust him with our lives, living in his leading.

We will all die. Some will sing with Frank Sinatra, about the way they lived – 'I did it my way'. The blessed of the Lord will sing 'I did it *his* way'. He created us; he redeemed us. Is there any better to entrust with our lives and our destinies?

Noting the departure of many of his disciples, Jesus asked of those closest to him, 'Will you go too?' Peter replies, 'To whom should we go? You have the words of eternal life.' He had a wonderful way of putting things!

We as carers are not much different from

those we care for. The difference is merely a few years. The same challenges face us all; how to make sense of our living and our dying? And how to live in the light of it?

As carers, we have been called – one way or another – into the practical loving of others. It isn't an easy calling, and many of us came to it kicking and screaming. But it carries the blessing of God, for, through learning to love, we start to see the nature of love more clearly, and the nature of sacrifice. And, if we will open our ears and our hearts, we will sense God closely with us – for he will draw close to those who love sacrificially. Service in the right spirit carries his 'Amen'.

We will understand sacrifice better, and we will know our imperfections more clearly (they always come into focus when we are under pressure!). So we will see the sacrifice of Christ for us more easily, and, knowing our imperfections, we will understand our need of Christ better.

One day there will be a glorious reuniting of those who love Christ, and trust him as redeemer. You will probably live longer than the one you care for. But there will be an end to all things, and a glorious re-union where none need care as once they did. There will come a time when all the pain and tears will be swallowed up in the love of the lamb of God, Jesus Christ. So let us encourage one another! And may God bless you mightily in your caring.

REDEMPTION
GLIMPSED

*May the God of hope fill you with all joy and peace in believing,
so that you may abound in hope by the power of the Holy Spirit.*

Romans 15.13

Since the very beginning, loving Father,
your realities have been breaking through.
You commanded light to shine in the first darkness
and in the coming of Jesus, your glorious word,
you made sure the darkness shall not overcome.
Through him, the way, the truth and the life,
you have given us a glimpse of your very self.

We praise you, for through your Holy Spirit
you inspired and sent Jesus to give sight to the blind.
We thank you for all the insights and understandings
you have given through the prophets and into our hearts
– all the glimpses of your brightness and glory.
But on the dark and painful days, in the dreary times,
we confess it is so hard to grasp and trust the truth.

*'My dear children, do not fear: am I not the one who created
you, the Lord who formed you? I have redeemed you;
I have called you by name; you are mine.'*
Isaiah 43.1 (paraphrase)

Thank you, Father, your word breaks through;
we need it as we care for those in danger or doubt,
in disease or despair – all for whom hope is thin,
over whom the darkness of death looms heavy.

'When you pass through the waters, I will be with you;
and through the rivers: they shall not overwhelm you.
When you walk through fire you shall not be burned,
and the flame shall not consume you.
For I am the Lord your God,
the Holy one of Israel, your Saviour.'
Isaiah 43.2

Yes! You have offered salvation, to give us hope.
Despite everything, in Jesus we see death on the Cross
turned into victory, new life and the hope of glory.
Though we may groan inwardly, Lord, grant us
to wait hopefully for the redemption of our bodies.
Though we may not see, let glimpses of your glory,
like rays of your sunlight breaking out of the clouds,
lighten both our days and our darknesses with hope.
Then may we be strengthened, comforted, cared for,
by the sound of your love – for your word says it all.

'Remember these things, my people, my beloved.
I formed you; you are my servants.
I called you; you will not be forgotten by me.
I have swept away your transgressions like a cloud,
and your sins like mist; return to me, for I have redeemed you.'
Isaiah 44.21, 22

Also by the same authors and published by Canterbury Press

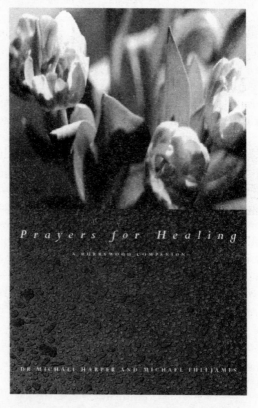

Prayers for Healing is a support for all affected by illness and disease, either in themselves or a loved one. Prayers and readings for morning and evening for 31 days reflect on a wide range of the bewildering emotions that are experienced. The authors have accompanied many in their journey through this unfamiliar and often frightening time, and here they offer their experience and wisdom gained in ministering to those who seek God's healing.

INFORMATION ABOUT BURRSWOOD

Burrswood Christian Hospital and Place of Healing was founded some 50 years ago by the late Dorothy Kerin in fulfilment of a commission from God, 'to heal the sick, comfort the sorrowing and give faith to the faithless'. The community is dedicated to bringing together Christ's healing ministry and orthodox medical care. It is recognized as a centre of excellence and experience in this field.

At the heart of Burrswood is the Church where public healing services are offered. It is integrated with a 35-bed registered hospital, 16-bed guesthouse, hydrotherapy pool, bookshop and tearoom set in a 225-acre country estate on the edge of Ashdown Forest. Many who come for a short hospital stay are enabled to do so irrespective of their means.

People find God's healing power at work through skilled nursing, medical expertise, prayer ministry and counselling. The aim is to keep the love of Christ at the heart of true whole-person care and to be a sign of the kingdom of God in a hurting world. Stillness and beauty provide space for the Holy Spirit's transforming work in every area of life.

Burrswood
Groombridge
Tunbridge Wells
Kent, TN3 9PY

General enquiries: tel. 01892 863637
Enquiries about staying as a guest or admission as a patient:
tel. 01892 863818

www.burrswood.org.uk